Outline of Clinical Diagnosis in the Horse

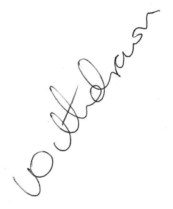

Outline of Clinical Diagnosis in the Horse ·

P. J. N. Pinsent BVSc, FRCVS
Formerly Senior Lecturer in Large Animal Medicine,
University of Bristol, UK

WRIGHT
London   Boston   Singapore   Sydney   Toronto   Wellington

Wright
is an imprint of Butterworth Scientific

 PART OF REED INTERNATIONAL P.L.C.

First published 1990

© Butterworth & Co. (Publishers) Ltd, 1990

British Library Cataloguing in Publication Data

Pinsent, P. J. N.
 Outline of clinical diagnosis in the horse.
 1. Livestock: Horses. Veterinary aspects
 I. Title   II. Series
 636.1089

ISBN 0-7236-0959-4

Library of Congress Cataloging in Publication Data

Pinsent, P. J. N.
 Outline of clinical diagnosis in the horse/P. J. N. Pinsent.
   p.   cm.
 Includes bibliographical references (p.
 ISBN 0-7236-0959-4:
 1. Horses—Diseases—Diagnosis.   I. Title.
 SF951.P39   1990
 636.1'0896—dc20

Composition by Genesis Typesetting, Laser Quay, Rochester, Kent
Printed and bound by Hartnolls Ltd, Bodmin, Cornwall

Contents

Preface   vii

1   Introduction   1

2   Abdominal pain   9

3   Clinical features of lymphosarcoma   31

4   Diarrhoea   39

5   The wasting horse   47

6   Hepatic disease   53

7   Diseases producing urinary symptoms   61

8   Respiratory disease – the coughing horse   65

9   Respiratory disease – the dyspnoeic horse   75

10 Dysphagia – difficulty in swallowing   81

11 Nasal discharge   87

12 Salivation   91

13 Allergic and anaphylactic conditions   93

14 Muscular problems   97

15 Lameness   103

16 Skin diseases   111

17 The udder   119

18 Peracute diseases, sudden death and 'found dead'
    syndromes   121

19 Pyrexia of unknown origin   125

20 Diseases producing nervous symptoms   129

21 The eye   137

22   The heart   143

23   Diseases of the foal   151

24   The laboratory   167

25   Special diagnostic procedures   179

Further reading   187

Index   189

Preface

In recent years, a considerable number of books have been written dealing with the medicine and surgery of the horse. This species has become increasingly important, not only to the specialist equine practice, but also to the farm animal practice, and particularly to the small animal practice in suburban areas, where the pony and riding horse population has increased so markedly. A number of these practices may have no interest in the horse. Many however would very much like to deal with the horse and pony work in their own area, but are deterred by a lack of confidence in their approach to the horse and its owner, and in their equine diagnostic technique. Such practices may well join the BEVA, and read the textbooks now plentifully available, but this apprehension about the equine approach often remains.

This book is intended primarily for the student, the new graduate, and the non-equine veterinarian seeking to become proficient in the handling of the increasing volume of equine work now available to him. If it proves to be of any interest to the specialist equine practitioner, that will be bonus indeed!

To my wife Connie, and my children Jill, Jim, John and Catherine

1 Introduction

The clinical attitude
The clinician's approach to the clinical case

The clinical attitude

The veterinary surgeon must develop certain special attributes in relation to his patient, and owners. He must be inquisitive, questioning, and observant. Everything going on around the horse must be noticed, and, if possible, explained. He must be critical in the true meaning of the word.

He will spend his life diagnosing disease, and must remember that, as disease is deviation from health, and as health is normality, then disease is simply deviation from normality. If he is to recognize the deviations from normal which constitute disease, then he must know the normal. The student, or the veterinary surgeon, not familiar with the horse must take the time and trouble to learn the normal. He must also realize that there is not just one normal in the equine species. For normality is relative, not absolute. It is relative to breed, age, type of work, management, environment, etc.

The veterinary surgeon must consider the environment as critically as he does the patient. Is it suitable for this particular horse? Does it predispose to, or even cause, the abnormality present? Does it cause stress? One must remember that the owner and his helpers are a very important part of the patient's environment, and may play a large part in the disease process. They, equally with, or perhaps even more than, other environmental factors, merit critical assessment. Are they competent? What do they know about stable management, pasture management, nutrition, and so on? Can they ride? Are they really interested in the welfare of their horse or pony? Is their equine knowledge sufficient to make their account credible? What do they really want? Have they contributed to the disease process? The owners merit critical study for they are inextricably involved with their animals, and one cannot consider one without the other. In the evaluation of an equine problem, the owner may be more important than the horse.

The clinician's approach to the clinical case

The important diagnostic principles are as follows:

(1) Be systematic.
(2) Adopt a routine which suits you, and stick to it.
(3) Take nothing on trust.
(4) Be continually self-critical; assess your attitudes and techniques, and keep up to date.

Consider always:

(1) Is there a problem?
(2) If so, define it.
(3) Having defined it, what is best done about it?

There is no magic about clinical diagnosis. It depends upon care, patience, thoroughness, method, and logical routine, a routine of examination which covers all the likely eventualities. Once having evolved such a procedure, there should be no short cuts without good reason, and however cursory some sections of the examination, for various reasons, may have to be, no step should be omitted without careful consideration.

Every clinical examination starts with the owner's complaint.

The owner's complaint

This should include *the type of horse*, including its sex and age, and *the main presenting syndrome*. A brief word on the severity and the duration of the problem may also be helpful. The owner's complaint is usually received by a secretary or receptionist and it is vital that she obtains enough information to allow you to assess the differential possibilities leading from the main presenting syndrome, and the urgency, or otherwise, of the case.

There are a limited number of main presenting syndromes, and the clinician soon makes out and learns differential lists for each of them. Include in those lists only the important and *common* differential conditions, for common things occur commonly; that is why they are common. Learn and know the common things. Do not worry about rare or bizarre possibilities, for you may never meet them.

Examples of important *main presenting syndromes* in the horse are:

• Chronic weight loss
• Chronic cough
• Chronic diarrhoea
• Abdominal pain (colic)
• Lethargy and poor performance
  etc.

On the way to see the horse, the veterinary surgeon considers his differential list. He may be able to narrow it down as he drives. For example, chronic pulmonary disease is unlikely to occur in a pony on good grazing in the spring; hyperlipaemia is very likely in a pregnant Shetland mare, but unlikely in a fit Thoroughbred in reasonable work; strongylosis is relatively unlikely in a housed hunter in the winter months, but is very likely in a riding school horse kept among many other horses on relatively bare pasture.

So the clinician considers his differential list against the time of the year, the horse's age, breed and type of work; the type of management, and the owner's skill, or otherwise, in equine matters. The patterns of disease among his own clients in his own practice become very familiar to a veterinary surgeon, and it may well be that he will arrive at the client's premises with his diagnosis at least half formed. Life becomes very much more difficult when one finds oneself dealing with strange clients in an unfamiliar background.

So the veterinary surgeon often arrives at the stable at least half way to a diagnosis. Such a diagnosis will be adaptable, not dogmatic, a *working hypothesis*, to be confirmed or refuted, but it is quite remarkable how often this hypothesis stands up to the test of full clinical examination.

History

History is all important, the foundation of diagnosis, and without it one is nowhere. *Immediate history* is the story of the present illness, *past history* includes anything in the horse's earlier life which might be relevant, e.g. did the horse cough when stabled last winter, and did the cough disappear when he was turned out to grass last spring, only to reappear recently when housed and fed hay again.

Group history may be very important in that adverse nutritional or managemental factors in a riding school or racing stable may have affected many horses to some degree, and be very relevant to the illness of the present patient.

History taking is an art in itself. It does not come naturally, but needs constant practice. After a few pleasant introductory words questioning can begin while on the way to the horse, which may be approached, but unless absolutely necessary, should not be disturbed. Look. Check the owner's statements mentally by reference to the animal and its surroundings. Do not hurry him at first; let him talk, then ask your questions, checking his statements, and following a routine which suits you. You are not wasting time, for you are, meanwhile, carrying out the next two stages in the clinical routine. Do not ask leading questions in an attempt to save time, for they often produce inaccurate answers. Human nature being what it is, the owner may either agree with you because he thinks he ought to, or disagree because he is contrasuggestive.

It is wise to study the owner or groom – is he reliable? Is he telling the truth? Is he covering up negligent management? Is he guessing? Does he know anything about horses? Every clinician must be interested in the human animal; after all, it is the owner whom you serve, advise, encourage, or console. In a way, the owner is more your patient than his horse. Admittedly, owners seldom falsify their story, but beware the guilty one, the bombastic one, the one who knows it all, and particularly the one involved in the sale of the affected animal.

Description

A formal description is not infrequently obligatory in the examination of a horse, e.g. as part of an examination for health or insurance, or during a vaccination procedure. But it is always useful to describe an equine patient mentally, for yourself, while you are taking the history. It is always potentially dangerous to be unaware of the exact nature of the horse under examination, as it may lead to loss of face in discussion of the case, and occasionally, even to serious error.

Preliminary inspection

Like the description, this inspection (*note* inspection, not examination) takes practically no time and may be carried out during history taking. Don't touch. Don't disturb. Stand well back. Get the horse in your mind's eye. Put the picture in its frame. You are looking for the deviations from normality which constitute disease, so it is worth stressing, once again, that *you must know the normal. Remember*, that if you frighten the horse, or excite it unduly, abnormalities will appear due to fear or annoyance. The minutiae which might have given a diagnostic lead may well be masked.

During the preliminary inspection, you should note the horse's condition, vigour, demeanour, respiratory patterns, appetite, faecal passage and type, response to the environment and so on.

Preliminary examination

Now you can approach and handle the horse, but it is essential to move quietly and with as little fuss as possible. This stage of the examination includes the rate and character of the pulse, the temperature, and a check on skin, eye, and mucous membranes. Pulse rate and character are very important in the examination of a horse, probably more important than in any other domestic species, and pulse rate increases very rapidly in an apprehensive or irritated horse. However quiet your approach, it is always wise to delay the pulse count until the patient is used to the feel of your fingers and the pulse rate has obviously slowed as much as it is going to.

By the end of the preliminary examination, the clinician may well have reached a diagnosis. He will, at least, probably be aware of the system involved. If so, he may need only to confirm his views by examination of that system, and by checking out the other systems quickly, even mentally. Nevertheless, the diagnosis may still be in doubt, and he will then need to carry out a systematic examination. So far, his procedure will have taken little more than a few minutes, but should a full systematic examination become necessary, the case becomes much more time consuming.

Systematic examination

This includes all the manual and instrumental techniques necessary as part of such an examination, even including, in some cases, surgical intervention. The veterinary surgeon, according to his training and inclination, may interpret the word *systematic* as meaning *thorough*, starting at the nose and finishing at the tail, or he may interpret *systematic* as meaning *system by system*, in which case he will have a mental list of the systems or sections which should be examined so that he can tick them off mentally when he is satisfied.

There is much to be said for adopting the second routine. It enables one to examine first the system or disease section which seems most likely from the preliminary evidence. Should the provisional diagnosis be confirmed then much time will be saved, for the check of the remaining systems to make sure that there is no other disease or lesion present will probably be reasonably brief. If, however, there is no provisional diagnosis in mind at the beginning of the systematic examination, then the veterinary surgeon may decide the order in which he carries it out. It is convenient to start with the most commonly affected systems, and to proceed, as necessary, to the less important.

A logical list of systems for examination is as follows:

• Circulatory system

- Respiratory system
- Digestive system
- Liver
- Locomotory system
- Skin
- Sense organs
- Lymphatic system
- Urinary system
- Genital system
- Nervous system
- Udder
- Parasite problems
- Metabolic problems
- Allergies

Obviously, the last three headings on this list of fifteen are not systems as such; they are, nevertheless, very important disease groups which may logically be considered as entities on the clinician's list.

Laboratory examinations

These are very important in the horse today, particularly in the diagnosis of liver disease, muscle disease, loss of weight, lethargy and poor performance, all common problems in the horse. Also, their use in the horse is not so likely to be ruled out by considerations of cost as in the farm animals.

Nevertheless, the clinician should never become slave to the laboratory. Laboratory investigation is intended to confirm or refute the provisional diagnosis (working hypothesis) already in his mind. Clinical examination comes first. Laboratory tests performed at random and out of context are likely to be misleading, irrelevant and confusing. They are always expensive. But if used logically and critically, they are often very helpful indeed.

Laboratory investigations include:

- Haematology
- Biochemistry
- Bacteriology
- Parasitology
- Serology
- Biopsy (histology) of tissues or fluids
  and finally:
- Necropsy

Even after full examination, one may not have a complete diagnosis. There should, however, be sufficient evidence to form a provisional diagnosis, a working hypothesis, which will allow the veterinary surgeon to embark upon a logical course of treatment. He must be prepared to use his commonsense, form a working programme even on insufficient evidence, have enough confidence to carry the owner with him, and enough adaptability to modify the programme tactfully if, and when, new evidence appears.

The owner, of course, is much more interested in *prognosis*, than *diagnosis*. Will his horse get better? and equally important, will it be capable of full work again? Is it going to cost a great deal? and will it be a long time before normality is regained?

2 Abdominal pain

The approach to the 'colic' case
The abdominal catastrophe
The sites of 'colic'
  Gastric colic
  Intestinal colic
    Spasmodic
    Tympanitic
    Impactive
Chronic colics – the chronic abdomen
Diseases simulating abdominal pain

Abdominal pain in the horse is, by common usage, referred to as colic. It may occur as an acute short-term syndrome, or as a low-grade chronic manifestation. In fact, colic means pain in the stomach or gut, rather than in the abdomen as a whole, but since abdominal pain, apart from that of parturition, is nearly always alimentary, there is no real objection to adopting the common usage.

Colic is not a disease, nor is it a diagnosis. It is merely a state of affairs, a syndrome, which indicates that the horse has pain in its stomach or gut. It is a syndrome common to many specific and differing conditions affecting the equine abdomen. When one observes this symptom, the diagnostic chain is just beginning. What is causing the colic? What is wrong with the horse?

It might even be wise to forget the term 'colic', and to think and speak instead of the *acute abdominal conditions of the horse*. This might encourage us to remember, when we next attend a horse with an acute abdomen, that the diagnostic chain is only just beginning, and that we must follow an orderly diagnostic procedure which will do three things:

(1) Differentiate from painful conditions unconnected with gut – the 'false colics'

Examples include parturition; dystokia, particularly uterine torsion; retained membranes; pleurisy; laminitis; azoturia; urolithiasis; and distension of a deep wound with pus.

Scrotal hernia may be included in this group for although it involves gut, the seat of pain is outside the abdomen, and its presence, or otherwise, should always be checked in an entire horse showing apparent abdominal pain. It might seem unbelieveable that conditions such as pleurisy, laminitis, azoturia, and even parturition should be confused with colic, but such confusion is a regular occurrence among inexperienced clinicians, and there are very few clinicians who can say, with confidence, that they have never made such a mistake, even if only transiently.

(2) Differentiate from general systemic diseases which include alimentary tract pain as part of a wider syndrome

Examples include grass sickness, anthrax, the early stages of salmonellosis, purpura, acute enteritis, arsenic poisoning, and the overeating of certain cereals, e.g. wheat.

It is worth stressing that certain diseases producing nervous signs, e.g. hepatic encephalopathy and hypocalcaemia, although, as far as we are aware causing no significant pain, may easily be confused with the acute colics.

(3) Having confirmed the presence of a true colic, arrive at an accurate diagnosis of the cause

The whole procedure must be orderly and routine in nature, no stage in the diagnostic process being left out without careful consideration. Let us consider our diagnostic approach to a colic case:

(a) *Treat every case on its merits. They are all different.*
(b) *Calm the owners.* This is vitally important. Colic has marked emotive effects upon owners and bystanders. It tends to produce over-anxiety, confusion and even panic in owners and attendants. The clinician must, whatever his inner feelings, appear calm, confident and imperturbable. If your own doubts or anxiety are obvious to the owner, the whole situation tends to get out of hand.
(c) *Pay attention to the horse's comfort and safety – check the potential hazards of the immediate environment* – a garage half full of old bicycles, garden tools, and mowing machines is a far from ideal place to treat colic. Make sure, as far as possible, that there is ample bedding, preferably non-edible, and that there are no objects such as buckets, mangers, etc., which can cause injury to the patient.
(d) *Watch quietly for a little,* before giving analgesics. The general symptoms of 'colic', i.e. digestive tract pain, are shown to a greater or lesser extent in all types of acute abdomen. Variations in severity, duration, and localization of the site of greatest pain intensity, are important aids to the correct diagnosis.

So, *stand back and look* – but not for too long.

(e) *Then relieve pain* – this is a vital part of the management of every colic case. Once the behaviour pattern has been noted, there can be *no* justification for allowing pain to continue. Pain leads to anxiety, exhaustion, injury, and may well predispose to unfavourable complications. Pain, in fact, helps to kill. It is quite unnecessary, so why allow it?

Why carry out the traditional and obsolete routine of keeping the patient on its feet, walking it endlessly, causing it further exhaustion, when it could be resting peacefully. It will not roll if there is no pain, not that the act of rolling is particularly harmful other than by causing injury and allowing the horse to become cast. There is no convincing evidence that rolling leads to the abdominal catastrophe, except, just possibly, in cases involving gross intestinal tympany.

The clinician of today has a number of analgesic drugs available from which he may select according to the clinical signs and severity. Pethidine, at a dosage rate of 2–5 mg/kg, given intramuscularly, gives very useful analgesia in most cases. It is important not to underdose. Many clinicians tend to keep to the bottom end of the dosage range – no harm will come of using the higher permitted dosages. It is inadvisable to give pethidine in muscles of the neck for there may be painful reactions, and a horse with an acutely painful neck is a problem even after the colicky pain has long disappeared. Pethidine should not be given intravenously, and the clinician must remember to maintain the scheduled drugs book accurately and promptly.

The analgesic action of pethidine is relatively transient, and, for many years, acepromazine (ACP) was used to support or enhance the effect of pethidine, or to alternate with pethidine in longstanding cases. But while pethidine has no serious contraindications, ACP may diminish peristalsis, and must not be used in a crisis situation lest the peripheral vasodilatation associated with its use should enhance shock. It is also true that the behavioural depression associated with ACP may mislead owner or clinician in their assessment of the horse's recovery.

In cases where there are signs of gut spasm, or where gut is tensely tympanitic, the mixture of hyoscine (spasmolytic) and metamizole (analgesic) produced by Crown Chemicals as Buscopan may be very effective. It may be given by intramuscular or intravenous routes in dosages of 20–30 ml.

An excellent analgesic is the non-steroidal anti-inflammatory drug flunixin meglamine (Finadyne) which, given by the intravenous or intramuscular routes at 1 ml/45 kg (1 ml/100 lb), is extremely effective and very rapidly so. Its very effectiveness is almost a disadvantage, for the improvement in demeanour is so spectacular in many cases that the owner may well believe that the horse is normal, when, in fact, serious abdominal lesions are present. It is therefore necessary for the clinician to satisfy himself that the pulse rate and character have returned to, and remained, normal, before he relaxes.

So relieve pain – in many cases of 'colic' nothing else is needed. In benign colics (i.e. those in which no abdominal crisis or catastrophe has occurred) such as spasmodic colic, relief of pain is all that is necessary, for recovery will ensue before the pain factor reappears. In simple tympanitic colics, analgesia plus antizymotics, and in simple colonic impactions, analgesia plus lubricants, will suffice.

Fortunately, the majority of 'colic' cases fall into these benign groups, and will recover, provided that the clinician uses a little commonsense, withholds food until recovery is complete, reintroduces it very gradually in bran mash form, adheres to proper clinical procedures and remembers the maxim 'Physician, do no harm!'

If, then, most colics are benign (spasmodic, tympanitic, or mildly impactive) and will recover as long as we do nothing stupid, what are we looking for when we commence a full clinical examination of the colicky horse, a straightforward procedure once we have achieved satisfactory analgesia, however impossible it seemed previously?

We are looking for the non-benign – the abdominal crisis or catastrophe, the case in which severe circulatory and organic damage has occurred, which cannot recover unless surgery is succesfully performed, and which, if surgery is, for one reason or another, withheld, will die miserably unless euthanasia is carried out.

Once we have decided that the case is, or is not, a case of abdominal catastrophe, then the most important decision has been made, and the rest of the diagnostic procedure can run smoothly on. Tension disappears – we know what to do. We are in charge.

Accurate diagnosis of the specific lesion in equine colic may be difficult, even impossible, but diagnosis of the catastrophic, as opposed to the benign, is relatively straightforward. And that is what matters!

There are reasonably clear criteria to follow. Learn them, trust them, and colic immediately loses its terrors.

Let us, now, consider the criteria to be assessed during the initial inspection, and during the full clinical examination, which may suggest the abdominal catastrophe.

Pulse rate and character

The pulse is, without doubt, the most important factor in the assessment of the colic case. Without knowledge of the pulse rate and character, *no* proper assessment can be made. *While the pulse rate is normal, nothing dangerous is happening,* even if it rises sharply to 50 or even 60 per minute during spasms of pain. As long as it falls to normal as soon as the pain has ceased, there is, as yet, nothing to fear. *We are not concerned by a pulse rate of 50 per minute.* Even between 50 and 60 per minute, although we may feel uneasy, there is still no overriding cause for worry, for surgery, or for euthanasia. *A rate of 60–80 per minute does give rise to concern, particularly if the rate stays high during analgesia.* Such a pulse, rising in rate, getting weaker, is depressingly significant. Circulatory damage is occurring, organic lesions are present. There are ischaemic areas of gut.

A pulse of 80+ is prognostically very grave indeed, especially if weak and compressible, and one will be particularly worried if the rate remains high or climbs higher in spite of the horse appearing to be in less pain. Toxic and necrotic changes are occurring. You have very little time.

Temperature is of little, or no, importance, save that a subnormal temperature associated with a rising pulse rate probably means that the terminal phase is imminent.

Pain

One is always worried when pain is continuously severe even under full analgesic dosage. One is even more worried when pain decreases, but the horse, instead of brightening, becomes dull and more depressed. If, meanwhile, the pulse rate rises, the position is grave indeed.

Mucous membranes

The state of the *conjunctival mucous membranes* is of great importance. While they are relatively normal in colour and appearance, there is unlikely to be severe circulatory damage. *But* the development of a deep brick red colour or a dirty somewhat jaundiced colour (with injected vessels) is a grave prognostic sign.

The respiratory pattern may be important

As circulatory damage, toxic changes and shock develop, respiration becomes rapid and jerky in nature. Sighing respirations also suggest a grave prognosis, while respirations which sound like a child sobbing may well indicate a rapidly developing peritonitis. *But notice* the accelerated respirations of that rarity – the *diaphragmatic hernia* – they may be heaving and laboured rather than rapid and jerky.

Generalized muscular tremors

These also have a grave significance.

Abdominal examination per rectum is all important

This is so important, in fact, that it is arguable that failure to carry out a rectal examination in a 'colic' case might amount to negligence. The procedure may be difficult and even dangerous in the animal in acute abdominal pain, but after satisfactory analgesia and sedation, it should, normally, not cause too much · difficulty.

There is no need, here, to discuss the interpretation of rectal examination in detail, for it is dealt with by Dr J. G. Greatorex in an excellent paper in the *Equine Veterinary Journal.*

In general, a relaxed and flaccid abdomen with ample room for manual movement is unlikely to be the site of a critical lesion. One must search for: solid masses, e.g. lymphosarcomas, enteroliths, etc., remembering that some solid masses, e.g. the impacted pelvic flexure, may be relatively benign; acute pain sites; indications of mechanical and circulatory obstruction, e.g. tense loops of gut distended with fluid and gas, tight and uncomfortable, displaced backwards towards the pelvis and upwards to the abdominal roof, allowing little, or no, room for the hand to move.

To aid one's assessment of the abdominal state, paracentesis may easily be carried out as described by Bach and Ricketts (1974), but the clinician may find that, in emergency situations, he seldom obtains unequivocal results unless there is purulent exudate or food material in the abdomen – not a very common finding. Laboratory examination of the paracentesis sample, possible in less severe cases, may be much more informative.

Faecal passage

Information regarding the movement of faeces is vital. If faeces are passed regularly, it is unlikely that there is organic or circulatory damage consequent upon actual obstruction. Even if faeces are passed in small quantities relatively infrequently, critically severe organic damage is unlikely, even if the pulse rate is somewhat raised.

But such signs may indicate the presence of a more or less localized gut wall lesion or lesions. Examples of such lesions are areas damaged by strongyle ischaemia; discrete 'lumps' of lymphosarcoma; diffuse lymphosarcomatous lesions involving a considerable length of gut; granulomatous enteritis; abscesses in the gut wall due to foreign bodies, or in adjacent lymph nodes due to 'strangles'; and terminal ileal hypertrophy.

Of these possibilities, strongyle (redworm) ischaemia is the most likely.

Gut wall lesions produce a low-grade, or sometimes acutely recurring, type of colic, which is usually noticeably worse after food, as a result of ischaemic, neoplastic or inflammatory lesions interfering with peristalsis. It is worth remembering that subacute impaction of the pelvic flexure, and very chronic grass sickness may produce a similar clinical picture. Such cases are most unlikely to present the signs of abdominal catastrophe. Any surgery carried out is likely to be *elective*, for the criteria which *demand* surgery are unlikely to be met.

It is worth remembering that faeces may pass from bowel distal to a complete obstruction of small intestine for some 8–10 hours after obstruction has occurred. The clinician, expecting that a complete obstruction would result in a complete cessation of faecal passage, may be misled and withhold surgery in the belief that the lesion is a gut wall lesion and that there is no abdominal catastrophe.

It is worth remembering that the frequent passage of flatus without any faeces appearing usually indicates an almost total obstruction.

Gastric filling, belching, 'vomiting'

It is almost as important to pass the stomach tube as it is to perform rectal examination, although the procedure may be far from easy until analgesia and/or sedation have been properly accomplished.

Passage of a tube may be of particular importance when there is distension of the anterior abdomen, when fluid has appeared at the nostril, or when belching frequently occurs.

The presence of large quantities of fluid and gas in the stomach indicate that:

(1) Acute grass disease may be present, in which case there will
be other signs.

(2) Primary gastric distension and tympany have occurred, in
which case, large volumes of gas and/or fluid will escape and
the patient will feel better.

(3) *There is an acute obstruction of the small intestine* – when the
prognosis will be very grave indeed.

The tube not only aids diagnosis as indicated, but also
decompresses the stomach prior to casting, anaesthesia and
surgery. It also allows the administration of fluids and
lubricants. Do not, however, give fluids or lubricants orally in
cases where passage of the tube has demonstrated a fluid-filled
stomach. You will only make things worse.

Laboratory aids to the assessment of the critical case

(1) Packed cell volume (PCV) and total serum protein are useful
guides to haemoconcentration. A PCV of 55% is very
worrying: 60% + very grave: 65% probably terminal.

(2) Blood urea level and *serum chloride* level may also be useful.
Serum chloride levels below 90 mequiv./l indicate electrolyte
loss.

(3) Blood pH and *lactate* levels help to assess the degree of
acidosis.

The practice laboratory may well provide PCV, serum
chloride, and lactate levels. Even if PCV is the only level
available in a night emergency, the information is well worth
having.

The horse in abdominal crisis develops haemoconcentration,
electrolyte and fluid loss, toxaemia, acidosis and shock.
Laboratory help, as indicated, can be invaluable in assessing
whether, and to what degree, these complications have
developed.

Having considered the criteria described, we may still have no
specific diagnosis. However we do know that there is something
very wrong, very difficult, that the prognosis is extremely grave.
We have diagnosed the abdominal catastrophe. If we trust our criteria
and follow their lead, we now have only two choices – we must
opt either for surgery or euthanasia. There is no other choice,
and there must be no more delay, for there is no more time.

What types of lesion are we likely to find in the abdominal

catastrophe case, either at laparotomy or post-mortem examination? The following is not an exhaustive list:

(1) Intussusception:
  (a) Small intestine alone.
  (b) Small intestine into caecum.
  (c) Caecum invaginated into colon.
  Many such cases adopt a trestle table attitude with legs wide apart and back dipped.
(2) Gastric torsion.
(3) Hernia through a mesenteric tear, or through the epiploic foramen. Diaphragmatic hernia.
(4) Volvulus or twist – often of the left ventral colon.
(5) Neoplasia – usually lymphosarcoma.
(6) Abscess in gut wall.
(7) Foreign body in wall of small gut – usually a nail or piece of wire.
(8) Foreign body in lumen of gut – usually an enterolith.
(9) Strangulation of small gut by the stalk of a lipoma.
(10) Torsion of gut on common mesentery.
(11) Submucosal haematoma of colon.
(12) Mesenteric abscess.
(13) Many manifestations of verminous strongyle infestation, varying from patchy ischaemia with fibrous tags and haemorrhages of the gut wall, to complete necrosis of several feet of gut: necrosis and perforation of the caecal tip, or even a very extensive paralytic ileus. In spite of a better understanding by owners of the control of redworm, and the availability of anthelmintics effective against migrating larval forms, parasitic gut damage is still a major factor in abdominal disease in the grazing horse.

The redworm is important not only in the classical verminous lesions, e.g. necrosis of the gut wall consequent upon arterial lesions, but also as a subclinical ischaemic factor interfering with intestinal motility due to oxygen impairment. Such interference may well dispose to impactive colic, while much spasmodic colic, and many cases of recurrent acute colic may well be associated with larval passage from the gut wall to produce lesions of arteritis in the enteric vessels.

If strongyles became extinct, colic might become a relative rarity. Unfortunately, in these days of overcrowded pony populations in which the major diseases are due to malnutrition and ignorance, the redworm would seem to have a secure future.

Care must be taken to avoid misdiagnosing grass sickness and the acute enteric conditions as abdominal catastrophies requiring immediate surgery. These conditions include anthrax, acute salmonellosis, other forms of acute enteritis, purpura haemorrhagica, cereal over-eating, particularly wheat, and even organophosphorus poisoning.

Peracute and acute grass sickness

These conditions may easily be misdiagnosed as acute colic crises, particularly in cases which are not quite typical. Confusion may be aggravated, in some cases, by a history of a colic attack 2 or 3 weeks previously, and then vague malaise, until the present attack suddenly supervened. There is usually distension of the stomach and small intestine, with as much as a threefold increase in volume of contents. There may be painful regurgitation of slimy green fluid stomach contents down the nose. The patient cannot swallow and attempts so to do result in water and grass-stained fluid appearing at the nostrils and wetting the upper lip.

The rectum is usually empty, its mucous membrane feeling peculiarly tacky on rectal examination. The colon, however, may contain varying amounts of stodgy material, simulating an impaction but with much less volume. There is no gut movement, and no faeces are passed. There may be slight tympany behind the last ribs, particularly on the left. Temperature is in normal range, but the pulse rate is characteristically 70+ per minute. There is abdominal pain, but not so much as one would expect from the pulse rate.

Patchy sweating is particularly prominent behind the elbows and in front of the stifles, while muscular tremors, visible over a wide area, are most marked at the same sites.

In cases not showing significant regurgitation. it is very easy to believe that one is dealing with an acute small intestine obstruction, with small gut and stomach full of fluid. Haematology and biochemistry will show the massive dehydration of blood and tissues, but there are no satisfactory diagnostic tests in life for grass sickness.

There is atony of gut from oesophagus to rectum inclusive, but no characteristic gut lesions develop. Endoscopy may reveal linear ulceration of the oesophageal mucosa, particularly in the lower third, but this is not a constant finding, and is more likely to be present when the horse has been stomach tubed. Lateral radiography after oral barium administration, using image intensification, usually shows marked incoordination of oesophageal movement, with delay in passage of contents into the stomach, dilatation of the oesophagus at various sites, and pooling of contents at the diaphragm. These tests are not helpful to the veterinary surgeon in field practice, and the truth is that it is still necessary to carry out laparotomy on some cases to demonstrate that there is no abdominal catastrophe. As soon as one feels beyond reasonable doubt that a case is one of grass sickness, it should, of course, be destroyed, but complete confirmation is still not possible until expertly performed histology of the coeliaco-mesenteric and stellate ganglia has demonstrated the characteristic neuronal degeneration. The fact that the highest incidence occurs in April and May in pastured horses from 2 to 7 years of age may be suggestive in a particular case, but can never be confirmatory.

Anthrax

This is fortunately rare in the horse in this country, and may also be confusing. There is usually, but not always, an initial high temperature, which may reach 106°F (41°C). This level drops as the disease progresses and by the time veterinary assistance is called it may be normal, or even subnormal. Pulse rate is always high, and tends to get higher as the disease progresses. The horse looks ill and very dull, and will not eat. Respiratory rate is rapid. Colicky pain and behaviour appear, and tense hot swellings caused by inflammatory exudate and oedema develop on the neck, throat and chest, causing respiratory difficulty. There may well be similar swellings of the prepuce or the mammary gland.

There is an acute enteritis, although diarrhoea may be relatively scanty with blood contamination. In advanced cases, blood may trickle from the anus. Death may result from septicaemia, or from asphyxia and toxaemia before septicaemia occurs. Thus, there may be no organisms in a blood smear. Occasionally, no head and neck swellings are present. Death usually occurs by the third day at the latest.

The post-mortem picture shows an acute and usually haemorrhagic enteritis, with blood-stained gelatinous swellings at the throat and at other sites of swelling. There may, or may not, be signs of septicaemia, and the spleen may, or may not, be enlarged.

Acute forms of enteritis

Acute forms of enteritis – particularly salmonellosis – may be very confusing. In recent years, salmonellosis has become relatively common in the horse. It seems that many horses are salmonella carriers, and the disease becomes clinical in times of stress, e.g. fatigue, transport, surgery, or coincidental disease, usually respiratory infections. It is particularly likely to appear in a clinical form if the horse is treated with oxytetracyclines or other antibiotic drugs excreted in the bile, for the antibiotic destroys the susceptible organisms in the gut, and allows the salmonella organisms which the horse is carrying to take over. It is possible that colitis X is, in fact, salmonellosis, triggered off by stress in a young carrier horse.

Salmonella typhimurium is the common type found in the horse, but *S. indiana*, *S. newport* and *S. enteritidis* also occur.

The important thing to remember is that although temperature may be markedly raised initially, it tends to fall quite dramatically as the disease progresses and may easily become normal, or even subnormal. Meanwhile, the pulse rate becomes progressively faster and may easily reach 100+ per minute. The horse is very depressed and stands still with head hanging. Bowel sounds are very slight at first, and initially there is quite marked abdominal discomfort without diarrhoea. As soon as diarrhoea occurs, bowel sounds become louder and pain ceases. In the early stages of this disease, there is usually a very low total white cell count with neutropenia, and this may be very useful diagnostically.

A similar story of abdominal pain with bowel stasis, followed by severe diarrhoea and cessation of pain, may occur in horses which have overeaten on wheat. Here, however, there will be no initial temperature rise, the diarrhoeic faeces often contain wheat grains, and laminitis may occur very early in the course of the disease.

Organophosphorus poisoning

This may well be confusing, but usually causes significant salivation, and scanty diarrhoea, as well as significant abdominal pain.

Purpura

A typical case of purpura in which the massive urticarial plaques, and haemorrhages of mucous membranes, are less pronounced than usual, may cause occasional confusion.

Always remember to examine the inguinal region of an entire with colic, and to suspect hypocalcaemia if a lactating mare shows colic-like symptoms with excitement, ataxia, sweating, collapse and muscular spasms. In an immediately preparturient mare, do not forget to check for uterine torsion which may be anterior to the cervix. A mare passing her placenta may show quite acute abdominal pain.

Some cases of azoturia, and many of rhabdomyolysis, may simulate colic. In theory, it should be easy to distinguish muscular pain from abdominal pain, but, in practice, it is not always so. Even acute laminitis can cause difficulty at first, while many veterinary surgeons will admit to having mistaken the initial dry stages of pleurisy for colic, only to realize their mistake when the exudative stages appear and a painful disease becomes a dyspnoeic one.

Fortunately, the abdominal catastrophes constitute a minority of the colic cases seen in practice. Most cases are 'benign' and fall into the following categories:

Gastric colic

The equine stomach, because of its small size, is readily susceptible to overdistension:

(1) *Distension with food, i.e. impaction* – due to overfeeding on grain with an insufficient water supply. This is a rarity today.
(2) *Distension with fluid, i.e. dilatation* – rare, apart from grass sickness, and obstruction of the small intestine which of course constitutes an abdominal crisis.
(3) *Distension with gas, i.e. tympany* – the result of the fermentation of succulents. This is the least uncommon form today. But it is probable that, as in the bovine abomasum, there is a primary inertia, possibly due to nutrition, possibly due to a primary lesion, as, for example, lymphosarcoma of the pyloric area. Tympany in its own right will cause considerable discomfort, with left-sided and anteriorly situated tympany, belching, and regurgitation of a mixture of fluid and gas. Such symptoms call for the immediate passage of a stomach tube, which will confirm the diagnosis and treat the condition at the same time.
   Unfortunately, gaseous dilatation (tympany) can easily progress to torsion, when the symptoms immediately become much more severe. The animal tends to take up a

dog-sitting position to avoid the pressure of the distended stomach on the diaphragm. There may be dyspnoea; the pain is acute; there is no gas in the rectum; the spleen may be pushed so far back that it is easily felt on the left side at rectal examination. It may be much more difficult now to pass a tube into the stomach, but every effort must be made so to do.

Intestinal colic

Spasmodic colic

As the name suggests, this condition is due to violent, irregular, incoordinate, peristaltic movements. There is, in fact, a segmental spasm of the small intestine. There is usually, also, a degree of intestinal tympany. The condition seems to be associated with fatigue, and with irregular and improper feeding. Horses which bolt their food are more susceptible. Nervous and anxious horses also may be more prone to attacks. The syndrome has been described as a neuromuscular disorder involving vagal excitability, but there is also some evidence that strongyle activity may have a part to play.

The clinical picture is of intermittent attacks of acute pain – rolling, crouching, sweating, stamping and kicking at the belly. During attacks, the pulse rate may rise to 50 per minute, but rapidly falls back to normal as the attack passes off after a comparatively few minutes. Temperature remains normal throughout. There are often very loud borborygmi associated with the most acute pain. No faeces are passed, but there are no vascular signs. Membranes remain normal, and between attacks the horse is bright and may even attempt to eat. Very often there are several such attacks, each one less spectacular than the one preceding it, and then the horse becomes normal again.

Flatulent or tympanitic colic

Excessive fermentation with severe tympany occurs in the large colon following greedy feeding on lucerne, clover, even grass cuttings, and sometimes fermenting grain. There may be a primary colonic atony – possibly as a result of strongyle damage. There is usually very well marked and resonant abdominal distension. There may be gas in the rectum. Loud borborygmi are audible. These sounds may quieten when the gut becomes very tense. Pain is severe and continuous, causing crouching, sweating, stamping, kicking at the belly and rolling.

As a result of the massive tympany, the large intestine becomes very unstable, and volvulus (twist or torsion) may supervene, usually involving the left ventral or left dorsal large colon, producing an abdominal catastrophe. The large colon kinking on itself strangulates the mesenteric vessels leading to necrosis, toxaemia and death.

Nevertheless, most cases of flatulent colic respond well to analgesics, spasmolytics, and antizymotics such as medicinal oil of turpentine.

Intestinal impaction (food impaction)

This affects the large colon, particularly the pelvic flexure, occasionally the other flexures, and rarely the small colon or caecum.

These colonic food impactions are traditionally stated to be due to faulty dentition, lack of water, and indigestible foodstuffs, e.g. straw and coarse hay. Such impactions often occur soon after the horse is brought from pasture into stables and a hard food regimen. Abnormal peristaltic movement may well be a primary factor, with local areas of atony, often resulting from verminous thrombosis. It is interesting that a number of cases subjected to laprotomy after failure to respond to normal treatment show clear evidence of ischaemic change in areas of the colonic wall, although the colon at that point is neither tense enough, nor its content hard enough, to believe that it could have become impacted in a normal gut.

Subacute impaction of the pelvic flexure of the large colon – the most common of the colonic impactions

It may take several days to develop fully, with progressively fewer faeces, getting harder and smaller until they cease altogether. There is low-grade dull pain, periodic in nature. The horse eats a little and drinks a little, except during more painful phases. It crouches, looks round at its abdomen, lifts its hindlegs alternately, and lies down a lot. It tends to adopt the urinating position, and this can lead to a misdiagnosis of urethral obstruction.

There may, in fact, be slight straining movements, and the tail may be carried a little high. There is very little, if any, abdominal sound. Frequent yawning occurs, which may cause confusion with liver disease, and the lips may be lifted back in a smiling position.

The pulse rate rises to slightly above normal. Rectal examination confirms the diagnosis, showing an impacted pelvic flexure and left ventral colon. The flexure may be on the pelvic floor or at the pelvic brim.

Treatment with analgesics, if necessary, and large volumes of liquid paraffin, or liquid paraffin/saline mixtures, combined with the withholding of all food, except small wet bran mashes, and the rectal manipulation of the impacted areas will be successful, even if tedious, in practically all cases. Neglected cases slowly deteriorate. The pain becomes continuous and more severe. The pulse rate rises progressively. The membranes get dirty and eventually jaundiced. Bilirubin and AST (aspartate aminotransferase) levels rise markedly. Eventually, necrosis of the gut wall, toxaemia and death will supervene, usually after a week or more of illness.

Impactions of the other flexures, or the terminal portion of the large colon

These are more painful. Pain is more continuous, and there may be a build up of gas behind the obstructing mass. Diagnosis is more difficult, for it is not always possible to detect and identify the site of obstruction by rectal examination. The pulse rate may rise to 50 per minute, but there are no signs of vascular interference, nor of shock.

Impaction of the small colon

This is rare, but can be very serious. Pain is continuous and acute. The impaction is usually very hard, and difficult to treat with fluids and lubricants. Some clinicians believe that an enema may reach the small colon and be useful in treating impaction. The small colon is considerably narrower than the terminal part of the fourth colon which immediately precedes it. Impaction usually occurs at this point of narrowing and may be felt on rectal examination as a very hard tubular mass extending posteriorly on the medial side of the caecum high in the abdomen.

Enteroliths

An enterolith is a calculus which develops in one of the sacculations of the large colon of the stabled horse and may remain there, symptomless, for years. If it becomes dislodged, as may happen when, after some years, the horse is turned to grass, it usually impacts in the first part of the small colon and causes continuous acute pain as severe as in small intestine obstruction.

In these days of the pastured horse, enterolith impaction is fortunately very rare.

Impaction of the caecum

This is also very rare, and probably occurs as the result of abnormal function of the caecal-colonic orifice. It may be that verminous damage is once again implicated. The condition develops very slowly over some weeks, with mild low-grade pain. The horse may eat a little and pass some faeces for a number of days before the faeces becomes scanty and cow-like. It spends much time lying down dully with its muzzle resting on the floor ahead of it, or round to its flank. Eventually, the caecal content builds up to a dense hard mass, which may be very difficult to treat by normal methods, and may necessitate elective surgery. The pulse rate remains in the normal range until, eventually, necrosis of the caecal wall occurs followed by toxaemia and eventually death. Diagnosis by rectal examination is reasonably straightforward, the caecum entirely filling the right side of the abdomen extending downwards and backwards from the abdominal roof in the lumbar region.

Occasionally, intussusception of the last part of the ileum into the caecum occurs. The clinical picture is initially similar to that of impaction, but it is virtually impossible to feel the abnormality by rectal examination. Eventually necrosis, toxaemia, gangrene and death occur. Diagnosis is only really possible on the basis of probability, confirmed by laparotomy.

Impaction of the small intestine

It is worth mentioning the acutely painful and fatal impaction of the small intestine known as sand colic. Traditionally, this occurred in Army horses on active service in the desert, but it is occasionally seen nowadays in ponies grazing, often picketed, on sand dunes with sparse grass. These cases are usually diagnosed on probability, taking the environment into consideration. They are very difficult to treat by conservative means, i.e. lubricants and fluids, and surgery may be necessary.

Schedule of procedure for management of subacute colonic pelvic flexure impaction cases

(1) Full clinical and laboratory examination.
(2) Place on non-edible bedding.
(3) Initial analgesics, if necessary.
(4) Give 0.5–1 gal. (2–4.5 litres) liquid paraffin and 0.5–1 gal. (2–4.5 litres) 0.5 N saline orally b.i.d. until faeces are soft and paraffin stained and impaction has disappeared on rectal examination.
(5) Water *ad libitum*, but no food for first 12 hours.
(6) Then a *small* wet bran mash twice daily and nothing else.
(7) Worm with wide-spectrum anthelmintics.
(8) Maintain on this regimen for 6 days until faeces are very wet.
(9) If during this period significant pain develops, then re-assess case – ?laparotomy or more liquid paraffin and saline.
(10) On seventh day, unless (9) has supervened, introduce hay very slowly and give drier mashes. If no pain, then increase and work slowly back to normal diet and regimen.
(11) If introduction of solid food (hay) produces further episodes of pain and recurrence of impaction, then consider *surgery* – exploratory laparotomy.

'Chronic colics' – the chronic abdomen

On the whole, the acute abdomen does not provide too much difficulty provided the clinician sticks to the rules. Many clinicians find much more worry in the management of the low-grade intermittent or recurrent colic case, which may go on for days, weeks, or even months, with progressive, if gradual, weight loss.

Are there any rules for these cases?

What are the most likely causes?

Most such cases have gut wall lesions – not, obviously, causing complete obstructions, but involving thickened, ischaemic, fibrosed, or otherwise damaged gut walls producing partial obstruction, or possibly just improper, irregular, peristalsis which slows down the rate of passage of ingesta. Some faeces are passed, but they are scanty and usually hard. Temperature and pulse are generally in normal range unless, or until, complications appear. Appetite is poor, and there is usually pain some 10 minutes after feeding. The most likely causes are:

(1) Pelvic flexure impaction is often, in part, a gut wall lesion. The initial lesion may be a worm damaged gut wall which leads to impaction at the flexure.

(2) Terminal ileal hypertrophe – a condition in which the walls of the terminal ileum become grossly thickened. May develop into an acute syndrome, diagnosed and treated at laparotomy.

(3) Chronic grass sickness – a clinical picture differing considerably from the acute forms. The primary feature is loss of weight over many days or even weeks. The horse is tucked up, herring gutted, with its back arched and its tail clamped between its legs. It may stand with all feet fairly close together like an elephant on a tub. Eventually, it assumes the appearance of an emaciated greyhound.

Respirations are slow, with sighing or snoring sounds. The penis is relaxed, there may be muscle tremors, and slight patchy sweating, particularly behind the elbows and in front of the stifles.

Appetite is poor, but the animal usually eats a little, preferably grass, and ingestion is followed in a few minutes by accentuated abdominal discomfort. The patient may then paddle, look around at its flanks, or even roll sluggishly. There is difficulty in swallowing, particularly water, and some grass-stained water may seep down the nostrils and wet the upper lip.

Haematological and biochemical parameters may have adjusted themselves, and may be more or less in normal range. Chloride levels, however, are usually low, and urea levels nearly always high.

(4) Obstructive lymphosarcomatous 'lumps' in the abdomen, often in gut wall, or in lymph nodes adjacent to the gut. These lumps are usually palpable on rectal examination.

(5) Low-grade diffuse peritonitis-affected visceral peritoneum.

(6) Gut wall abscessation (foreign body) or strangles abscesses pressing on gut wall.

(7) Migrating strongyle larvae causing ischaemic areas and irregular peristalsis.

(8) Malabsorption syndromes due to granulomatous enteritis of the small intestine, or diffuse lymphosarcoma of the wall of the small intestine.

The last four conditions are often difficult to differentiate (see Chapter 5).

Probably strongylosis is the most common cause of gut wall lesions – most chronic abdomens are linked with redworm infestation.

Procedure for diagnostic and therapeutic management of chronic colic cases in which the diagnosis is initially in doubt (see also Chapter 5)

(1) Full clinical and laboratory examination.
(2) Place on non-edible bedding.
(3) Initial analgesics, if necessary.
(4) Water *ad libitum*, but no food for first 12 hours.
(5) Then *small* wet bran mash twice daily *and nothing else*. These horses are best treated in hospital, away from the owner.
(6) Worm with wide-spectrum anthelmintic.
(7) Maintain on this regimen for 6 days until faeces are very wet.
(8) If, during this period, significant pain develops, then consult (10) below. However, this seldom happens unless the horse is allowed to eat solid food.
(9) On seventh day, introduce hay very slowly. If no pain, then increase and come slowly back on to normal diet and normal regimen.
(10) If introduction of solid food (hay) produces further episodes of pain, then consider:
   (a) Euthanasia.
   (b) Rest for further period and re-assessment.
   (c) Surgery – but remember that surgery may:
     (i)   show operable lesion,
     (ii) show inoperable lesion (destroy),
     or
     (iii) not show anything at all, which means either:
       • no lesion, *or*
       • you have missed it, in which case you may either: destroy, or bring animal round and start again.

Diseases simulating abdominal pain

When considering the diagnosis and differential diagnosis of colic (acute abdominal pain) we must remember that a number of diseases which produce convulsions, hyperactivity, dyspnoea, or nervous signs may well cause confusion and be misdiagnosed as colic.

Examples include:

- Hypocalcaemia (p. 130)
- Transit tetany (p. 130)
- Hepatic encephalopathy (p. 55)
- Polymyositis (p. 83)
- Botulism (p. 83)
- Uraemia (p. 62)
- Acute anaphylactic episodes – acute anaphylactic shock or acute allergic pulmonary disease (pp. 70 and 79)

Both the veterinary surgeon and the client are much more familiar with abdominal pain syndromes than with the conditions listed above. It is quite understandable that in difficult diagnostic situations the client calls the veterinary surgeon to a 'colic case', and the veterinary surgeon accepts the diagnosis because the other possibilities are considerably more obscure.

There is no magic in making a diagnosis from the list above. Do not hurry: watch quietly, even if the owner and his staff are apprehensive and on edge. Do not panic. Think. Take the time to obtain a full history and to ascertain the circumstances of the case and any relevant environmental factors. And while you are doing this watch the patient for the clinical minutiae. For example: hypocalcaemia cases will be mares and almost certainly have a foal at foot. Transit tetany cases may be ponies of either sex, or bigger mares in oestrus or lactating. They are, or have just been, in transit by road or rail; or have suffered some equally severe stress. The encephalopathy case may be jaundiced; will have been dull, depressed, and yawning for at least 12 hours and maybe more, and may have photosensitization lesions developing or white-skinned areas of face and muzzle. Polymyositis cases will have been choking, discharging grass and saliva via the nostrils, and will be becoming less and less able to stand. There will be myoglobinuria and often some degree of jaundice. Botulism cases are entirely relaxed; they become quietly weaker, and even when completely recumbent they lie quietly with a minimum of struggling. And so on. Gradually the case falls into its proper diagnostic compartment, and often with a minimum of handling.

References

Bach, L. G. and Ricketts, S. W. (1974) Paracentesis as an aid to the diagnosis of abdominal disease in the horse. *Equine Veterinary Journal*, **6** (3), 116

Greatorex, J. G. (1968) Rectal examination as an aid to the diagnosis of some medical conditions in the horse. *Equine Veterinary Journal*, **1** (1), 26.

3 Clinical features of lymphosarcoma

Abdominal
Thoracic
Generalized
Skin

It is probable that, setting aside skin and other superficial tumours, lymphosarcomatous lesions are the most common form of neoplasia met with in the horse.

It has been said, not infrequently, that the lesions of lymphosarcoma in the horse are so haphazardly arranged that no patterns exist. Fortunately for the clinician this is quite untrue. The clinical patterns of this disease are relatively clear cut and well defined, and experience suggests that the most important syndromes can be set out as follows:

(A) Abdominal
   (1) *Space-occupying lesions within the peritoneal cavity*, affecting lymph nodes, mesentery, omentum, and gut wall.
   (2) *Diffuse lesions affecting gut wall:*
      (a) Small intestine – producing a malabsorption syndrome.
      (b) Large intestine – producing diarrhoea.
(B) Thoracic lesions (mediastinal:thymic) – producing space-occupying masses in the chest, with thoracic effusion and dyspnoea.
(C) Generalized lymphosarcoma
   (1) Affecting bone marrow and blood.
   (2) Bilaterally symmetrical involvement of lymph nodes.
(D) Lymphosarcoma of the skin.

Abdominal

Space-occupying lesions within the peritoneal cavity

These usually involve, in the first instance, lymph nodes, mesentery and omentum, followed by spread to the gut wall, and possibly, eventually, to other abdominal organs, e.g. spleen, kidney and liver.

These lesions form the 'lumps and bumps', so-called, found at rectal exploration, and may occur at a number of sites within the abdominal cavity. They may achieve considerable size, but do not necessarily cause symptoms until they invade gut wall, unless, of course, they are placed so as to cause intermittent external pressure upon gut.

Normally, however, symptoms are associated with invasion of gut wall – the so-called 'gut wall colic' syndrome involving relatively low-grade intermittent pain particularly associated with the period following feeding.

One such case suffered intermittent relatively low-grade colic for a year, with episodes increasing in frequency and severity until eventually the horse suffered 'colicky' episodes at least once a day after feeding.

It is, of course, bulk food, rather than mashes or small feeds of grass, which cause pain. The *differential diagnosis* of 'gut wall colic' and, therefore, of this type of lymphosarcomatous lesion, includes a number of conditions, which give the clinician more problems in diagnosis, management and treatment than most of the acute abdominal crisis situations. They are:

(1) Terminal ileal hypertrophe – episodes tend to be acute.

(2) Chronic grass disease – behaves as a gut wall lesion – often shows some colonic impaction; can be very confusing, but usually causes slow and awkward swallowing, loss of abdominal volume, an 'elephant-on-tub' stance, pendulous penis, clamped-down tail, patchy sweating and muscle tremors. In particular, the pulse rate is 50–60 per minute, even when no pain is present.

(3) Obstructive lymphosarcomatous *'lumps'* acting by pressure alone.

(4) Gut wall abscessation – penetrating foreign body or strangles (rare).

(5) Migrating parasitic larvae – ischaemic areas.

(6) Malabsorption syndromes:

(a) Diffuse small intestine lymphosarcomas	Very difficult to
(b) Granulomatous enteritis	differentiate
(c) Diffuse low-grade peritonitis	clinically

The most common gut wall lesion is, of course, ischaemic, due to strongyle damage.

A useful diagnostic technique involves feeding small wet bran mashes, twice daily, and keeping the horse on an inedible bed. Practically all gut wall lesions cease to hurt *immediately* on this regimen, and one can then proceed to more detailed diagnostic work:

- Rectal exploration
- General demeanour
- Loss of weight
- Increasing anaemia
- High white cell picture with marked neutrophilia
- Paracentesis (Bach and Ricketts, 1974) – concentrated fluid may show lymphosarcomatous cells
- The more gut wall is involved, the lower the serum, albumin, and the greater the possibility of ventral oedema
  This gradation is important

One can progress steadily along a series of cases, starting with abdominal masses (lumps and bumps) and moving through cases with greater and greater gut wall involvement, until, eventually, one meets the case where there is diffuse involvement of the *mucous membrane and submucous tissues* of practically the whole of the gut with no other lesion save those in the associated lymph nodes and *with little, or no, involvement of the serous coat*. Thus, one now has a *malabsorption* syndrome, with minimal pain, due to a *diffuse infiltrating lymphosarcomatous takeover of the mucous membrane*. The following features should be looked for:

- If lesion is of small intestine, then the uptake of nutrients is involved
- Very low pain level ? imperceptible
- Fair appetite
- Ample faeces
- Loss of weight
- Low proteins
- Neutrophilia
- Anaemia
- Much ventral oedema – protein-losing enteropathy
- Temperature – normal. Pulse rate ? normal
- Concentrated paracentesis fluid may show lymphosarcomatous cells

It is very important to notice that, at post-mortem, the lesions of the mucous membrane may be almost imperceptible, and it is possible for an experienced equine pathologist to open the small intestine, examine it, visually, and by palpation throughout its length, and discard it as normal, only for the clinician, with faith in his tests, to retrieve it for histology and demonstrate practically 100% lymphosarcomatous involvement of mucous membranes.

In such cases of progressive weight loss with ventral oedema, *low proteins* and minimal or no pain, having cleared liver (sorbitol dehydrogenase, serum alkaline phosphatase and gamma glutamyl transferase) (for remember chronic liver damage is very important as a cause of chronic loss of weight) and kidney (very rare) then you must do *glucose uptake* (or xylose uptake) tests.

Obviously, *malabsorption with diffuse lymphosarcomatous infiltration* gives a nil glucose uptake. So, unfortunately, does the fascinating condition of *granulomatous enteritis*, which normally affects younger horses. And so may some cases of *diffuse serous peritonitis*, e.g. following colic with slight perforation and adhesions. But the end point is the same and post-mortem will differentiate.

Of course, diffuse lymphosarcoma of mucous membranes does not have to be confined to small gut. It can affect large gut – COLON. In which case, the malabsorption effect will affect water uptake and *chronic diarrhoea* will be the result.

Differential diagnosis now includes:

(1) Diffuse lymphosarcoma – progressive diarrhoea, loss of weight, electrolyte loss, slight abdominal pain, anaemia, neutrophilia, ventral oedema, and progressive ill health.
(2) Chronic salmonellosis – faeces sample should confirm.
(3) Chronic parasitic ulcerative colitis – very important in the grazing horse, but the horse is bright, eats, drinks and does not feel ill until the terminal stage. It may adapt and show clinical recovery.
(4) Avian tuberculosis of gut (ileo-caecal area) – behaves like Johne's disease in the cow.

It is possible for more than one of these diseases to be present in the same horse.

Cases may occur in which the last part of small intestine and the first part of large intestine are involved, *with partial malabsorption and some diarrhoea.*

Thoracic lesions: mediastinal – thymic

A fascinating and clear-cut syndrome, although often misdiagnosed when first seen. Occurs in horses from 2 to 7 years old. A surprisingly rapid course, which sometimes seems to be triggered by a recent (3–4 week previous) upper respiratory tract infection.

Symptoms include:

- Poor exercise tolerance
- Increased respiratory rate – abdominal lift – dyspnoea
- Occasional cough. Elbows out
- Stretched neck
- Anterior ventral oedema – sternum and thoracic inlet
- Swelling in jugular furrows at inlet – ? lymph node – ? tumour itself
- Corded jugulars and facial veins

- Accumulation of saliva in mouth with champing and attempts to swallow
- Normal temperature. Variable pulse. Loss of weight
- Anaemia
- Heart muffled but audible over wide area. May be murmur
- Fluid in chest – many litres, many white blood cells may be lymphoblasts
- Peritoneal fluid less, in volume, but similar in type

Diagnostic aids include:

- Obstruction to stomach tube
- Paracentesis
- X-ray
- Auscultation and percussion

N.B. There may be secondary hyperlipaemia.

The lesion is usually a *multilobar lymphosarcomatous mass in the mediastinum.*

Generalized lymphosarcoma

(1) Affecting bone marrow and blood vessels.
(2) Bilaterally symmetrical involvement of lymph nodes.

Affecting bone marrow and blood vessels

One case of generalized lymphosarcoma involving bone marrow and blood vessels with massive lymphocytosis showed the following clinical picture:

A 7-year-old Thoroughbred gelding with pyrexia, distension of tendon sheaths, and oedema of legs to stifle and elbow. Lethargic and dull. Weight loss.
Poor appetite. Pulse rate 60 per minute. Ventral oedema. Panting respirations. Anaemia (PCV 14.5%).
Weak. Wobbly. Haemorrhage from nostrils and injection sites.
White cells rose to 26 000 per mm^3 *with 99% variously aged lymphocyte cells.*

Post-mortem showed multiple haemorrhages, with peritoneal blood clots, and blood splashings in respiratory tract and heart.

Bone marrow – showed little else but immature lymphoid cells – blast cells.

Lung capillaries were packed with cancer cells.
Lymphosarcomatous changes in lymph nodes, spleen, liver, kidney, heart and lungs.

An *identical* case has recently been seen in a slightly older riding horse. *Identical* is not quite accurate, for the blood picture in this case showed 90% lymphocytes in a very *low* white cell count. But that was the position early on in the previous case.

Bilaterally symmetrical involvement of lymph nodes and lymphoid tissue

The occasional case shows bilateral protrusion of the eyeballs due to lymphosarcomatous masses in the orbits. There may be swellings of lymphoid tissue on face and neck, bilaterally symmetrical enlargement of superficial lymph nodes, neoplastic changes in most body organs and a marked lymphocytosis, with anaemia and weight loss.

Lymphosarcoma of skin

This is another relatively rare manifestation of lymphosarcomatous disease. Firm domed lumps varying in circumference from a 50 pence piece, to irregular masses several inches across, develop in irregular patterns over the skin of neck and body. Eventually, they may ulcerate. Definitive diagnosis must be by biopsy.

Reference

Bach, L. G. and Ricketts, S. W. (1974) Paracentesis as an aid to the diagnosis of abdominal disease in the horse. *Equine Veterinary Journal*, **6** (3), 116

4 Diarrhoea

Acute
  Superpurgation
  Anthrax
  Salmonellosis
  Clostridial enterotoxaemia and diarrhoea
  Complications of virus respiratory disease
  Purpura
  Organophosphorous poisoning
  Rhododendron poisoning
  Peritonitis
  Hyperlipaemia
  Cereal overeating
Chronic
  Nutrition
  Strongylus vulgaris
  Chronic parasitic ulcerative colitis
    (strongyle)
  Chronic parasitic colitis (trichonema)
  Diffuse colonic lymphosarcoma
  Granulomatous colitis
  Avian tuberculosis of the large gut
  Chronic salmonellosis
  Fungal infestation of gut
  Occasional cases of liver disease
  Rare cases of chronic grass disease
  Prolonged phenylbutazone therapy

Diarrhoea in the horse is fortunately not particularly common, but when it occurs it is always serious. The clinical picture may be either acute or chronic.

Acute diarrhoea

Superpurgation

The effect of drugs containing aloes derivatives – anthraquinones – which are particularly dangerous in Thoroughbreds. The anthraquinones were used extensively for the purgation (physicking) of horses, but are now more or less obsolete. Some horses showed very severe idiosyncratic reactions even to half doses, and suffered persistent acute diarrhoea, often tinged orange in colour, until dehydration and electrolyte loss became very serious.

Anthrax

Anthrax is relatively rare in the horse in Britain, and may well not appear as a septicaemic disease (cf. the cow). There is usually an initial temperature of 105–107°F (41–42°C), falling rapidly and becoming subnormal. There is abdominal pain, so that the disease requires differentiation from the acute colics, or acute forms of salmonellosis. There is acute haemorrhagic enteritis producing severe blood-stained diarrhoea. There are usually inflammatory swellings containing exudate and haemorrhage which appear around the throat and on the ventral and lateral parts of the neck and chest, but such swellings are not a constant finding. Death usually occurs in a few hours up to about 24 hours. The blood smear stained with polychrome methylene blue may not be confirmatory as many cases have not become septicaemic and exudate from the swellings should also be examined.

Salmonellosis

This has become much more important in the horse in the past 20 years. A number of *Salmonella* organisms occur including *typhimurium, enteritidis, newport* and *indiana*. The disease occurs in varying degrees of severity from the very acute to the chronic. It must be remembered that salmonellas are opportunistic organisms, much more likely to set up clinical disease in horses under stress, unduly fatigued, or recovering from major surgery. Coincidental illness, particularly respiratory infections are also an incitement to the disease. Equine hospitals are at particular risk – horses from distant areas arrive, and may include among their number salmonella carriers, which may, under stress, rapidly become acute cases, and infect other stressed patients which may also become clinical. Some horses become carriers without suffering from the clinical forms of the disease, but a stressed horse meeting the organism is much more likely to succumb. Infection builds up in a hospital and is difficult to eradicate. It is necessary to empty the hospital, carry out complete disinfection, and *then allow the premises to lie fallow for a month*. Such a procedure is very disruptive, and regular sampling from drains and corners, etc. must be carried out. The disease was at its worst in the 1970s, but is now, probably due to greater awareness, much less of a problem. Owners must be warned that a recovered acute case may remain an excretor for several months, and some chronic carriers remain so indefinitely.

This aspect of the disease can often be confusing. A horse with a very minor diarrhoea problem may be a chronic carrier, and positive faecal swabs may be misleading in such a case. One recent diarrhoeic pony was suffering from redworm infestation, avian tuberculosis, salmonellosis and colonic lymphosarcomatous infiltration, but it is likely that the parasites and the bacteria involved were all opportunists, the neoplastic change being primary.

Under the Zoonoses Order (1975) it is necessary for the laboratory isolating salmonella to report to the Environmental Health Officer, but it is wise for the clinician in change of the case to notify the Area Liaison Officer, usually at the local Veterinary Investigation Centre.

The acute form of the disease usually starts with a very sick horse with a temperature which may be as high as 106°F (41°C). It will be dull and depressed and hanging its head, with a totally miserable demeanour. There is low-grade abdominal pain. The acute diarrhoeic phase comes some hours later, and when this happens pain lessens. Occasionally blood and mucus are evident in the diarrhoea. The total white cell count and the neutrophil count are very low at this early stage – there may be as few as 1000 total white cells per cubic millimetre. The neutrophil percentage is also very low. This is a very useful diagnostic feature in the early stages of the disease. When the diarrhoea appears, the temperature begins to fall, the white cells rise, and the pulse becomes very fast and weak. Respirations are rapid and may become dyspnoeic. Dehydration and haemoconcentration supervene with a high packed cell volume (PCV). The mucous membranes become discoloured and the patient may go into severe shock. The condition affects all ages and may be so peracute that the horse dies before diarrhoea is seen, thus posing a difficult diagnostic problem requiring differentiation from acute colics, anthrax, and the clostridial enterotoxaemias.

On the other hand less acute pictures occur grading down to the chronic picture of diarrhoea, wasting, and occasional slight faecal blood. Diagnosis of these cases may not be easy, so it is imperative to culture faeces of any scouring horse for salmonella.

During the 1970s when equine salmonellosis became widespread it was some time before the profession became aware of its real nature. For some time it was believed to be an oxytetracycline toxicity, for it was not uncommon for sick horses treated with oxytetracyclines, then widely used in equine practice, to develop acute salmonellosis, for the antibiotic was excreted in the bile and removed the competing bacteria in the gut. The condition known as 'colitis X' was probably also acute salmonellosis, affecting as it did young horses which had been unduly stressed by fatigue. Some cases of 'colitis X' may have been clostridial enterotoxaemias which occasionally occur.

Acute post-mortem picture

Dehydration, subcutaneous congestion and haemorrhage. Gut lesions largely affect the large gut producing a dull reddish brown discolouration of the serosa of the caecum and colon, with congestion and haemorrhage of the mucosa. There may also be epicardial and myocardial haemorrhages.

Clostridial enterotoxaemia and diarrhoea

It is only recently that *Clostridium perfringens* (*welchii*) and *Cl. difficile* have been recognized as the aetiological factors in certain enterotoxaemic and diarrhoeic conditions in the horse. Symptoms are very acute with low-grade abdominal pain and a high temperature rapidly falling. Mucous membranes are discoloured, and there is dyspnoea. Haemoconcentration and shock occur. The horse may well die before diarrhoea occurs, i.e. in 24 hours or less, but if diarrhoea supervenes it is profuse, watery and blood stained. Definitive diagnosis is by the detection of clostridial toxins in the gut content, or by culture of the organisms themselves. Differential diagnosis – primarily salmonellosis.

Complications of influenza and other virus respiratory diseases

Secondary bacterial enteritis can occur in horses suffering from influenza – salmonellae among other organisms may be involved.

Purpura haemorrhagica

An acute anaphylactic condition traditionally regarded as an immune reaction to *Streptococcus equi*, but possibly a manifestation of any acute anaphylaxis. There is massive oedema of the head, neck and lower limbs, with oedematous plaques on the body. Haemorrhage of the gut occurs with abdominal pain and blood-stained diarrhoea. There may be fatal necrosis of the affected areas.

Organophosphorus poisoning

This can occur occasionally in the horse, causing abdominal pain, tremors, profuse salivation and diarrhoea. Muscular weakness, ataxia, attempts at vomiting, and a slow heart rate may also occur.

Rhododendron poisoning

Poisoning due to ingesting rhododendron occurs mostly in winter when snow interferes with grazing, or when pastures are scorched in a summer drought. The symptoms include salivation, vomiting, ataxia, low-grade abdominal pain and diarrhoea.

Peritonitis

For completeness it should be mentioned that a horse suffering from postoperative, and sometimes from other forms of peritonitis may develop a toxic scour – dark, sticky and not usually profuse.

Hyperlipaemia (hyperlipidaemia)

Usually this is seen in small fat ponies with an illness producing energy deficiency, exposed to deliberate dieting, or around the time of foaling. Signs include weight loss, depression, difficulties in prehension due to myopathy of the muscles of face and lips, profuse milky fat in the blood producing a creamy appearance, and a greasy fatty diarrhoea. Such animals have a grossly fatty liver which undergoes massive fat mobilization under energy deficiency stress.

Cereal overeating

Overeating on barley, and even more seriously on wheat, causes depression and abdominal discomfort, with raised pulse rate. The symptoms may suggest that the case fits one of the acute colic categories, but hopefully diarrhoea, often containing wheat or barley grains, will occur before laparotomy has been carried out. Acute laminitis is a not infrequent sequel to cereal overeating, and the feet must be checked twice daily.

Chronic diarrhoea

Nutrition

Can be caused by rank, wet spring grass. Excess of barley and particularly wheat produces very severe diarrhoea with acidosis which may even be fatal.

Strongylus vulgaris

The adults in the gut of the young horse cause weight loss and diarrhoea, with a high total white cell count, anaemia, and high β and α_2 globulins.

Chronic parasitic ulcerative colitis

This occurs as a result of a massive presence of *Strongylus vulgaris* larvae in the blood vessels of the colon wall, producing thrombosis of the vessels and ischaemic end point ulcers in the wall. Fibrosis of the gut wall leads to inability to absorb water, a major function of the equine colon. There is resultant diarrhoea and increased thirst, with weight loss, anaemia, ventral oedema and dehydration. It is common in this condition for the horse to pass portions of soft faeces in a considerable volume of faecal-coloured watery fluid, with the result that if the horse is at grass the owner does not realize the full extent of the diarrhoea, for the fluid soaks into the soil leaving only the soft faecal portions to be noticed. Serum albumin is low, beta globulins high, and the total white cell count is usually high with a neutrophilia.

The horse does not feel ill until a late stage in the disease for there are no systemic lesions beyond the gut wall. The position may alternate better/worse. The onset is insidious and progress slow; some patients are only slightly affected and some degree of compensation occurs leaving them bright and active, but poor thrivers, with faeces soft but not diarrhoeic.

Chronic parasitic colitis

Chronic parasitic colitis, often of a more severe nature, may be due to the presence of numbers of trichonema cysts in the colonic wall – the clinical picture is seen largely in the spring – much damage may be caused to the gut wall when the cysts erupt. The clinical picture then is acute, and eventually produces much fibrous change in the gut wall with resulting failure to absorb water. Such a case must have been grazing infected pasture the previous autumn.

Diffuse lymphosarcomatous infiltration of the wall of the large gut

This produces a water malabsorption and diarrhoea. The lesion is diffuse and only appreciable histologically, causing thirst and low-grade pain with low serum albumin, dehydration, and weight loss. There may be lymphosarcomatous cells in the peritoneal fluid, and there is usually leucocytosis and neutrophilia. Lymphosarcomatous infiltration of the wall of the small intestine, however, causes progresive weight loss, but no diarrhoea, for in this case the malabsorption relates to food, not water.

Granulomatous colitis

A chronic inflammatory and diffuse lesion of the colon wall, possibly an immune reaction. This condition also causes pain but somewhat more severe in nature than the lymphosarcomatous lesion previously described. There is thirst, loss of weight, and diarrhoea. This condition, like its counterpart in the small intestine, granulomatous enteritis, is rare in Britain.

Avian tuberculosis of the large gut

Avian tuberculosis can affect liver, spleen and lymph nodes, but in the large gut produces a diffuse lesion causing diarrhoea, dehydration and weight loss. The symptoms and the lesion itself resemble the picture in Johne's disease in cattle. Most equine avian infection seems to be derived from pheasants kept on the same farm or estate as the affected horse.

Chronic salmonellosis

Discussed previously on p. 41.

Fungal (aspergillus) growth in the gut

This can be the result of prolonged oral antibiotic therapy, which has often been given to treat a diarrhoeic condition already in existence, producing a stubbornly resistant diarrhoea.

Chronic liver disease

Very occasionally this produces diarrhoea. However, most liver disease is associated with varying degrees of constipation.

Very chronic grass disease

Occasional cases can develop a scanty diarrhoea.

Prolonged phenylbutazone therapy

In small ponies, e.g. Shetland and Welsh, this may lead to anaemia and diarrhoea developing.

5 The wasting horse

The approach to the wasting horse
Well or unwell: environment or disease
    Conditions causing persistent pain
    Conditions interfering with mastication or
      swallowing
    Conditions interfering with gut function
      (diarrhoeic and non-diarrhoeic)
    Chronic liver conditions
    Chronic kidney conditions
    Chronic heart conditions
    Miscellaneous conditions

'Wasting', 'Loss of condition', 'Abnormal thinness', whichever term you wish to use, is not a disease in itself. It is not a diagnosis, nor even really a symptom. It is merely a state of affairs.

Remember that we only describe a horse as a wasting horse if we cannot find an obvious cause for its loss of weight. You would not call a horse with a suppurating joint a case of loss of condition, although it certainly loses flesh very fast – you would call it a case of sepsis.

It follows, therefore, that when we finally classify a horse as a case of loss of condition, one or two states of affairs must hold good:

Either we have failed to detect the clinical signs and failed to obtain the laboratory data which should give us a lead as to the cause of the loss of weight, *and this is our failure.*

Or there are no clinical signs, nor abnormal laboratory data, in which case the horse is not ill, which means that the loss of condition is *environmental.*

This is the first decision we have to make – is this a *thin well* horse or a *thin ill* horse. That sounds ridiculous, but there is an important distinction, and every effort should be made at the outset to decide to which category your case belongs. If you are certain in your own mind that the loss of condition is environmental, then you must take a searching look at the environment for yourself. Put no trust in the owner's assessment of what constitutes enough food, or enough grass, etc., for their assessment may differ widely from yours.

Obviously, the most likely causes of loss of weight include:

- Insufficient food
- Insufficient grass
- The wrong sort of food
- Not enough water
- Too much work
- Irregular work in an unfit horse causing sweating and distress

It is sometimes regarded as useful confirmatory evidence in this type of case if the various laboratory tests you apply all give normal results – *but beware* – follow Herod's advice to Claudius – trust no one nor anything, particularly laboratory tests – a horse can die with a normal range of laboratory results.

From what we have said so far we must remember, in considering the thin unwell horse, that the clinical signs will be minutiae only. Therefore, we must examine the case minutely and meticulously.

It is very difficult to come to a diagnosis at one examination. Quite often, it is not the medical examination which yields results, but prolonged observation over a number of days. *Hospital observation is therefore all important.*

(1) It is very useful to know what happens to the horse when you feed it.
(2) It is very important to spend an hour or two or more leaning quietly over the box door and watching.

Prolonged undisturbed observation, and in some cases, *serial laboratory examination,* are very important. Obviously, in cases where clinical evidence may be slight, we are tempted to use laboratory aids, and because we don't know what we are looking for, we tend to run a wide range of laboratory tests in the hope that something may show up. This may provide very misleading results.

It is also expensive. All laboratory tests are expensive and overuse can add a great deal to the bill without giving much additional information. The use of serial laboratory tests, essential if one is to obtain a reliable picture of an ongoing disease process, has become prohibitive.

Few horses and practically no ponies justify a bill, easily built up, of £100 for laboratory tests, when they are suffering from a chronic wasting disease where the prognosis is inevitably poor. So, what one needs is a tidy routine laboratory procedure which will confirm, or refute, as far as possible, the more important conditions which cause loss of condition in the horse. We need a minimum of tests, and each test must be particularly related to specific disease conditions, reliable and cheap.

First, one must consider the most likely causes of 'loss of condition'.

Conditions causing persistent low-grade pain

For example:

(1) Bilateral forefoot lameness.
(2) Chronic brucellosis – low-grade discomfort, lethargy, cautious movement, stiffness, intermittent temperature, depression and loss of weight.

Conditions interfering with mastication and/or swallowing

(1) Teeth – very important – always check.
(2) Very chronic grass sickness. Peracute, acute, and subacute grass disease provide classical symptoms which draw

attention to themselves over and above any loss of condition. But mild cases of the chronic form may show, primarily, loss of condition over many days or even weeks. The pony may be tucked up and herring gutted with an arched back and the tail clamped down. The penis will be relaxed, there will be muscular tremors and patchy sweating, particularly behind the shoulders and in front of the stifle. Practically no faeces are passed, and any that are may be cow like. Such a pony will eat a little, preferably grass, with marked difficulty in swallowing. This difficulty may be more marked when attempting to drink and water may return down the nostrils. There is usually low-grade abdominal pain after eating.

Packed cell volume (PCV) is usually raised. Sorbitol dehydrogenase (SDH) and aspartate aminotransferase (AST) may be somewhat raised. Total serum protein values may be, but serum chloride will be, low. Blood urea is usually high.

(3) *Myopathies involving muscles of prehension* – ? low Se/vit. E often associated with hyperlipaemia and/or steatitis. Most ponies with hyperlipaemia, and many with steatitis, have an associated myopathy of the muscles of prehension. These ponies are inappetent, but they try to drink, without success. They can only splash their mouth and lips in the water, they cannot imbibe, and so no water comes down the nostrils. This is an important differential feature.

(4) *Pharyngeal paralysis following upper respiratory tract infections.* In mild cases, dysphagia may be low grade, water may come down the nose, food may be eaten very slowly, swallowing may be difficult and traces of food may appear at the nostrils.

Conditions interfering with intestinal function (absorption and/or motility)

Diarrhoeic

(1) *Nutritional* – e.g. wet and luscious grass.

(2) *Chronic salmonellosis* – has a low incidence in adults – causes weight loss, diarrhoea, and dehydration. There is no blood in the faeces, and the temperature is normal. The organism may be an exotic salmonella, e.g. *S. indiana*, and usually occurs in ponies already ill due to worm damage, gut lymphosarcoma, etc., i.e. the case is one of previously subclinical infection activated by stress.

(3) *Redworm.* First, the adult in the colon of the young animal causing loss of flesh, anaemia, dehydration and diarrhoea.

Secondly – very important – parasitic ulcerative colitis, due to gut wall damage in older ponies caused by migrating strongyles or encysted forms resulting in failure of water absorption.

(4) *Lymphosarcoma* diffusely affecting the colon wall – such cases usually show mild discomfort.

(5) *Avian tuberculosis* – some cases affect gut and show signs similar to Johne's disease in the cow. Note that avian tuberculosis may also affect liver, spleen and lymph nodes producing emaciation without diarrhoea.

Non-diarrhoeic

(1) *Damage due to migrating redworm larvae* – lesions of verminous arteritis, thrombus formation, and abscessation leading to ischaemic areas of gut and abnormal peristalsis. *Always low-grade pain.*

(2) *Lymphosarcoma* in diffuse arrangement along wall of small intestine – malabsorption syndrome – *low-grade discomfort* – particularly after food. A protein-losing enteropathy – ventral oedema – low serum albumin.

(3) *Granulomatous enteritis – low-grade discomfort* – particularly after food. Also a protein-losing enteropathy – there is often ventral oedema and low serum albumin.

(4) *Chronic grass disease – low-grade discomfort* – particularly after food.

(5) *Strangles abscessation* in mesenteric lymph nodes, etc.

(6) *Chronic peritonitis* – usually following colic and producing a diffuse arrangement of lesions along the peritoneal lining of the small gut. There may be an intermittent slight temperature rise.

(7) *Villous atrophy* – obscure aetiology.

Chronic liver conditions

There may well be ventral oedema associated with low serum albumin.

- Ragwort
- Chronic toxic change
- Senile cirrhosis
- Liver fluke

- Avian tuberculosis
- Chronic abscessation
- Biliary obstruction related to pancreatic lesions

Chronic kidney conditions

Very rare in horses, but one occasionally meets cases of *chronic interstitial nephritis* – senile changes, loss of weight, mouth ulcers, uraemic odour, uraemia, panting respiration, proteinuria.

Pyelonephritis – undulating temperature, loss of weight, oedema of ventral abdomen and legs. Rapid pulse, uraemia, blood, pus and debris in the urine.

Degenerative kidney changes associated with redworm damage to the kidney vessels. Kidney disease is relatively easily diagnosed in most cases by blood urea estimation, plus urine analysis. Chronic kidney conditions may also lead to low serum albumin conditions, and protein-losing enteropathy.

Chronic heart conditions

Heart lesions seem to cause loss of weight only when clinical cardiac congestive changes are present. (n.b. Systolic murmurs in many Thoroughbred foals are not significant.)

Miscellaneous causes

- Tuberculosis (bovine)
- Ectoparasites
    Lice
    Mange
- Bots
- Continual pruritis
    Allergic dermatitis
    Head flicking
- Excessive windsucking and flatulent colic
- Excessive sexual activity in mares
- Thyroid hypertrophe (adenoma?) in older horses
- Old age

So *plan* laboratory tests in relation to *gut and liver, with kidney a poor third.*

6 Hepatic disease

Acute
    Mild reversible
    Severe irreversible – acute hepatic failure
        Plant hepatotoxins
        Toxic factors
        Viruses
    Hepatic encephalopathy
    Blue-nose disease – photosensitization and
      encephalopathy
Secondary – hyperlipaemia
Chronic – cirrhosis
Pancreatic lesions causing biliary tract
    obstruction
    Cholelithiasis
    Jaundice
    Lethargy, anaemia, poor performance

Diseases of the liver are diagnostically difficult from the clinician's point of view. The liver has many functions and symptoms of disease vary depending upon the extent to which different hepatic functions are affected. It is not unreasonable to think of the liver as a number of organs combined within the same capsule. There is also much variation in the severity and extent of the pathological lesions of liver disease. Liver dysfunction is relatively common in horses, and may be classified as follows.

Acute liver disease

The acute case shows severe clinical signs, and has a guarded prognosis. From both clinical and pathological viewpoints the acute syndrome is divided into:

(1) *Mild reversible parenchymal cell damage,* and
(2) *Severe irreversible cell damage – acute hepatic failure.*

Acute cases tend to occur during the second part of the summer on into the autumn. They are due to:

(a) Many hepatotoxins in pasture plants, even plants as commonplace as red and white wild clovers. It is interesting that even ragwort, normally causing slowly progressive chronic liver damage, occasionally produces an acute case.
(b) A wide selection of other toxic factors.
(c) Several viruses. Viral hepatitis may be very severe, as was shown during the outbreak of serum jaundice which followed the use of infected prophylactic sera some 20 years ago. The clinical picture has a sudden severe onset. There is profound depression with long periods of dummy behaviour often spent standing with half-chewed hay hanging from the mouth. Very frequent yawning occurs requiring differentiation from the yawning seen in subacute impaction of the pelvic flexure of the colon, certain forms of meningitis and encephalitis. There is usually jaundice, although one has to be very careful in assessing jaundice in light-coloured horses, particularly in artificial light, as the colour of the sclera may suggest quite wrongly that jaundice is present. Many cases are constipated, and show low-grade abdominal discomfort. The urine tends to be concentrated and dark in colour.

In very severe cases hepatic encephalopathy develops. It

tends to occur in the severe irreversible form, and obviously suggests a very grave prognosis. It is due to faulty liver function allowing an excess of ammonia to develop in the circulation. Hyperammonaemia leads to encephalopathy causing ataxia, leaning on walls, head pressing, aimless and incoordinate wandering, followed by intense excitement during which it may become quite dangerous to approach or handle the horse. Eventually this phase is followed by collapse, coma and death.

Notice that a somewhat similar ataxia and wandering picture may occur in the terminal stages of uraemic disease, usually following irreversible acute renal failure.

In horses with acute liver damage, the liver may be unable to deal with the circulating phylloerythrin resulting from chlorophyll metabolism, and in horses with areas of non-pigmented or flesh-marked skin, photosensitization may occur. With very rare exceptions photosensitization in horses is an indication of liver disease. The non-pigmented and flesh-marked areas become acutely inflamed and may ooze serum. In a few days the affected skin becomes obviously dead and leathery and begins to separate from the adjoining pigmented skin. In fact the condition known as *blue-nose disease* is in all probability acute liver disease showing encephalopathy and photosensitization. It occurs in horses grazing during the summer months. Pasture hepatotoxins, mostly clovers, cause acute liver damage, and thus phylloerythrin passes through and reaches subcutaneous areas via the circulation. An inflammatory reaction takes place in the presence of sunlight, causing oedema of the muzzle, face, eyelids and occasionally other areas. White legs may be affected. The facial oedema becomes most severe over non-pigmented and flesh-marked areas, which become bluish (cyanotic) and ooze serum which forms crusts and scabs. If recovery occurs the skin of the muzzle sloughs and heals by granulation. Usually the horse becomes dull, depressed, and jaundiced, and then maniacal. The prognosis is always grave when encephalopathy is present. The severe acute form with its terminal encephalopathy is easy to confuse with meningitis, encephalitis, brain tumours such as psammoma, and an acute hepatic case with some abdominal discomfort followed by encephalopathy may easily be confused with colic.

Note the form of acute liver disease known as *serum jaundice*. A severe outbreak occurred some 20 years ago as a result of injecting grazing horses with influenza serum of equine origin.

It was originally believed to be an immune reaction to equine antiserum, but it is now generally accepted that it was a *viral hepatitis*, due to contamination of a large batch of antiserum. The condition showed all the signs of acute liver disease plus a terminal myoglobinuria due to an accompanying myopathy.

Secondary liver disease – hyperlipaemia

This bears some likeness in principle to ketosis in the cow. It is a response to energy starvation due to illness, to deliberate dieting in fat ponies, to toxic effects, or to pregnancy in small fat ponies, particularly Shetlands. Rapid mobilization of fat occurs producing extensive fatty change in the liver and usually in the kidneys as well, leading to 'choking' of the blood with triglyceride fats. It is part of the wide syndrome of defective fat metabolism in ponies, which includes steatitis and yellow fat disease as well as hyperlipaemia. If in doubt, look at the blood – let it settle – it will look obviously fatty. Shetlands are frequently affected, and may develop the disease in the absence of a primary lesion, purely from the stresses of late pregnancy and parturition.

It takes several days to reach the height of the disease. The pony is stiff, slow and dull. There are usually no faeces passed, but there is slight abdominal pain and definite muscle tremors. There may be slight jaundice. There is concomitant myopathy involving the muscles of prehension (possibly vitamin E and selenium are involved); the pony cannot pick up food or water; it splashes in its water. It has been suggested that the myopathy may be the primary lesion, and the hyperlipaemia secondary to the starvation so caused. Laminitis, worms, lymphosarcoma, or deliberate fasting, may all be primary syndromes. The pulse rate is 60–80, and the temperature in normal range. Constipation gives way to a scanty, greasy diarrhoea. Heavily pregnant mares are likely to abort, or foal early; the foal, even if alive, is likely to scour because the milk may contain a high level of triglyceride fats. Acidosis may occur causing rapid shallow respirations. Encephalopathy does not develop, but severe cardiac fatty change may provoke collapse. The mortality is 60–70%.

Chronic liver disease

This, effectively, means cirrhosis of the liver, and is usually due to ragwort poisoning. Other causes include liver fluke infestation, senile cirrhosis, chronic abscessation, reaction to on-going low-grade toxicity, and the 'recovery' phase after acute hepatic disease. Symptoms include insidious and progressive weight loss, anaemia, weakness, and eventually ataxia. Inappetence develops slowly, and there is a tendency to constipation although a sticky, scanty diarrhoea, occasionally associated with straining, may develop in the terminal stages. Ventral oedema occurs due to hypoalbuminaemia, and there is often some oedema around the face and neck, varying in distribution and extent. The temperature remains normal but the pulse rate may rise slowly. There is no obvious pain. Eventually signs of hepatic encephalopathy occur – yawning, head pressing, standing with food in mouth, great depression, low-grade mental aberration, followed by staggering, collapse, coma and death. Photosensitization is unusual in chronic liver disease: jaundice may occur but is much less common and less noticeable than in the acute syndrome. *Diagnosis* is aided if mental symptoms are present, but it is then usually too late to help. Absence of pain helps to differentiate from abdominal strongyle infestation, chronic grass disease, and abdominal lymphosarcoma. Ragwort is the most likely cause – search the fields and hay for it. Fluke infestation in horses is relatively rare and occurs largely in areas where there is heavy cattle infestation. Precautionary dosing may be wise. Avian tuberculosis of the liver may occur without gut involvement – diagnosis is very difficult. The tuberculin test may be helpful but is not easy to interpret in the horse.

A clinical picture to all intents and purposes indistinguishable from chronic cirrhotic change is due to:

Pancreatic lesions causing biliary tract obstruction

Eventually in this condition an exudative dermatitis of the coronets and lower legs develops – this sometimes occurs in hepatic cirrhosis, e.g. ragwort poisoning, and must make one suspicious of liver problems. A condition known as *chronic active hepatitis* does occur in horses, which look well, eat well and are apparently in good health but cannot maintain condition when put to work, even if the work load is light. They also become lethargic. Gamma glutamyl transferase (GGT) and serum alkaline phosphatase (SAP) are very high. Biopsy shows portal tracts with large numbers of inflammatory cells – neutrophils, macrophages, plasma cells and lymphocytes. There is an increase in portal fibrous tissue extending into the neighbouring parenchyma. The condition is certainly inflammatory and not primarily degenerative, but will lead to severe cirrhosis if ignored. It responds well to intensive steroid therapy; GGT and SAP fall; but even after several weeks of steroids and some months' rest some cases deteriorate when work begins again. If ignored, cirrhosis spreads, and these cases need as much as a year's rest, with a regular check on GGT, if they are to be useful again.

Notice that horses fed on propionic acid-treated hay in an attempt to avoid mouldy hay may develop mild hepatic dysfunction and become lethargic. Entires may show lack of libido.

For laboratory examination of hepatic disease see Chapter 24.

For biopsy method and BSP test techniques see Chapter 25.

Remember – very important – whatever else you do to treat a case of hepatic disease, it must be allowed complete rest.

Cholelithiasis (gallstones)

This syndrome is rare in the horse, which has no bladder. Stones do not form easily. Diagnosis is difficult. Symptoms include depression, and episodes of abdominal pain, at first transient and slight. The mucous membranes are congested. Temperature and pulse rate tend to rise during the course of the disease – jaundice develops. There may be ascites. Eventually hepatic encephalopathy supervenes. SAP, GGT and bilirubin all rise markedly, and sorbital dehydrogenase (SDH) and aspartate aminotransferase (AST) rise slightly. The disease is fatal.

Jaundice

Jaundice in the horse may cause the clinician considerable embarrassment. Many grey and chestnut horses appear slightly jaundiced if examined in artificial light. Also, there is always a tendency to diagnose hepatic disease in a jaundiced horse without full consideration. In fact many, if not most, cases of severe jaundice are due to causes other than primary liver dysfunction.

For example, marked jaundice may occur:

(1) In obstinate impactions of the pelvic flexure presumably due

to reabsorption and recycling of bile. Jaundice tends to develop in cases persisting for four or more days.

(2) In cases where very large haematomas have developed, as for example in steeplechasers or hunters which have hit the top of a solid jump with their sternum and developed a large haematoma of the brisket. Here again jaundice takes several days to develop.

(3) In acute polymyositis, which is seen occasionally in native ponies in marginal areas. There is severe myoglobinuria. Jaundice may be very pronounced in this condition.

(4) In leptospirosis – here haemoglobinuria may be very severe, but the first sign of the disease is often a faint yellowing of the sclera some 12 hours before any other symptom is apparent to the attendant.

Jaundice is also marked in cases of cholecystitis, viral (serum) hepatitis, acute irreversible hepatic failure, and is noticeable in many cases of ragwort poisoning, hyperlipaemia, and photo-sensitization.

Anaemia, lethargy and poor performance

These symptoms are seen relatively frequently in horses. The following circumstances are examples.

(1) Starvation and debilitating disease.
(2) Chronic liver damage.
(3) Chronic blood loss – generally due to strongyle parasitism (normochromic, normocytic).
(4) Neoplasia, particularly lymphosarcoma.
(5) Foleic acid deficiency (old, mouldy hay) (macrocytic).
(6) Iron deficiency – (microcytic) usually secondary to chronic haemorrhage, e.g. parasitism.
(7) Postviral debility – influenza or rhinopneumonitis – often associated with leucopenia, neutropenia, and relative lymphocytosis, especially if not rested properly.
(8) Red cell breakdown – e.g. haemoglobinuria – leptospirosis is a good example.

7 Diseases producing urinary symptoms

Pyelonephritis
Strongyle degeneration
Chronic interstitial nephritis
Acute renal failure
Cystitis
Urolithiasis
Redwater
   Haematuria
   Haemoglobinuria
   Myoglobinuria

Diseases of the urinary system are not common in the horse. Pathological examination frequently discloses lesions of the kidneys, but these are seldom extensive enough to cause clinical disease. Owners tend to worry unduly about renal disease, possibly because of the cloudy, turbid, and highly coloured appearance of quite normal equine urine. Equine urine should always be spun down or filtered before urine analysis is performed. Kidney conditions do, however, occur from time to time, and among them are:

Pyelonephritis

This causes an undulating temperature with raised pulse and weight loss. There are varying degrees of inappetence, oedema of the ventral abdomen and legs, and lethargy, with blood, pus and debris in the urine, and eventually uraemia. Diagnosis depends on urine analysis, blood urea estimation, and culture of urine to reveal the causal organisms, usually streptococci.

Degenerative changes

These are a result of strongyle larvae damaging the renal veins, producing massive swelling of the affected kidney, with considerable abdominal pain and haematoma. Ventral oedema may be present. It may be possible to palpate the enlarged kidney per rectum.

Chronic interstitial nephritis

A senile change occurring in very old horses, with weight loss, mouth ulcers, uraemia, uraemic odours, panting respirations and proteinuria. Urine is dilute and low in albumen. This is a picture of chronic renal failure.

Acute renal failure

This occasionally occurs secondary to toxic insults of various kinds, usually chemical (e.g. chlorinated hydrocarbons and certain weed-killers). Symptoms are acute. The horse will neither eat, nor drink. Urine is passed in very small quantities, if at all. Temperature is normal, but pulse rate is high. Urine may be concentrated and contain debris and casts. Blood urea rises rapidly and the nervous signs of uraemia appear. These include ataxia, aimless wandering, excitable behaviour, staggering and collapse. The prognosis is grave.

Cystitis

Cystitis occasionally occurs in horses, causing the passage of small quantities of urine frequently, sometimes with a tendency to straining. There may be a slightly raised temperature and some inappetence. There are blood cells and bacteria in the urine, with tissue debris.

The differential diagnosis of cystitis includes urolithiasis.

Urolithiasis

In this condition calculi may be present in the bladder or urethra. The mare, with a short and distensible urethra, seldom if ever develops urethral calculi, but cystic calculi in the mare often attain a considerable size. Even in the male, calculi are more common in the bladder than the urethra, but urethral calculi do occur. Cystic calculi may cause a somewhat stiff gait, and occasionally slight abdominal discomfort. A very small amount of urine is passed at any one time, and may contain blood. Diagnosis by rectal examination is usually straightforward when the bladder is empty, but in the mare the calculus can sometimes be touched with a finger in the urethra, and in both sexes a catheter can be tapped audibly against the calculus in the bladder. The urethral calculus in the gelding can often be diagnosed by passing a catheter. The bladder may be distended and this shows on rectal examination. Any urine passed will contain blood and debris, and the horse strains to pass it. There may be significant colicky pain, and the horse's stance suggests subacute impaction of the pelvic flexure of the large colon. It is, however, much more likely that the clinician will misdiagnose pelvic flexure impaction, believing it to be urethral impaction.

Differential diagnosis of 'redwater'

It is important to determine accurately whether red colouration of the urine is due to haematuria, haemoglobinuria or myoglobinuria, for each of these materials leads to a different group of diseases.

Haematuria

(1) Pyelonephritis.
(2) Strongyle damage to renal vessels.
(3) Cystitis.
(4) Urolithiasis – urethral calculi.

(5) Endocarditis – thrombosis in the renal vessels causing haemorrhage.
(6) Renal carcinoma – very rare – horse will be dull with a poor appetite. There may be pyrexia. There will probably be metastases in lung and liver. Rectal examination may help diagnosis.

Haemoglobinuria

(1) Equine infectious anaemia – only one episode has occurred in this country.
(2) Babesiasis – probably non-existent in this country.
(3) Haemolytic disease (iso-immunization) of the newborn foal.
(4) Autoimmune disease in the adult – very rare.
(5) Incompatible blood transfusion.
(6) Leptospirosis – a number of leptospiral serotypes affect horses, and a significant proportion of horses show leptospiral antibodies. Clinical cases, however, are relatively rare. Symptoms include pyrexia (106°F, 41°C), jaundice, acute anaemia, severe haemoglobinuria, abdominal discomfort, leucocytosis and neutrophilia.

Myoglobinuria

(1) Rhabdomyolysis – especially azoturia and polymyositis.
(2) Viral hepatitis – the form of viral hepatitis known as serum jaundice causes a terminal pigmentation of the urine which some authorities believe to be myoglobin rather than haemoglobin.

Differentiation between haematuria and haemoglobinuria is easily carried out:

(1) Centrifuge the urine sample. In haematuria the red cells settle quickly: in haemoglobinuria the colour remains diffuse, or
(2) Let the sample stand for half an hour. The result is as above, but not quite so clearly, or
(3) Examine the sample under the microscope: the presence or otherwise of large numbers of red cells will decide the issue.

However, deciding between haemoglobin and myoglobin in urine is much more difficult. Myoglobin looks much browner than haemoglobin, but biochemical analysis is necessary for certainty.

8 Respiratory disease – the coughing horse

Strangles
Rhinitis
Influenza
Rhinopneumonitis
Miscellaneous viruses
Chronic pulmonary disease
Pollen allergy
Parasitic bronchitis
Nasopharyngeal lymphoid hyperplasia

This is a very important differential group in the horse, which is, in most cases, a professional athlete.

Strangles

The justification for discussing strangles at this point is that, in its early stages, the symptoms include reduced appetite, a slight cough, and a serous nasal discharge, with an inflamed pharynx which sometimes makes swallowing difficult, and a raised temperature (103–105°F, 39.5–40.5°C). At this stage the symptoms may lead to an incorrect diagnosis of influenza, or rhinopneumonitis with subsequent embarrassment, and possibly errors in treatment. The serous nasal discharge, however, quickly becomes profuse, purulent and creamy white in colour. This material pours from both nostrils, and as the horse snorts, blows and shakes its head, it is distributed widely in the immediate environment. Culture of this pus produces *Streptococcus equi*.

There is a slight increase in the respiratory rate. Meanwhile the submandibular nodes become enlarged, hot and painful. They get bigger for several days, hard at first and then soft and fluctuating producing a large central oozing swelling denuded of hair with increasing skin discolouration. There is considerable peripheral oedema. In some 10–14 days from the onset of the disease the abscess ruptures discharging the same type of creamy white pus. Normally the temperature then falls rapidly, the horse rapidly feels better, recovers, and remains largely immune.

Complications and undesirable sequelae do, however, occasionally occur. Abscesses may occur in the subparotid lymph nodes, or in the retropharyngeal lymphoid tissue. Suppurative bronchopneumonia, or pus in the guttural pouches may occur. Abscesses in mediastinal and mesenteric lymph nodes may rupture to produce fatal suppurative pleurisy or peritonitis. Occasionally areas of cellulitis develop, especially over the face, throat and ventral neck. Rarely abscesses form in the brain, lungs, liver and kidney as a result of bacteraemic spread. These complications are known collectively as irregular or 'bastard' strangles. *The most dangerous sequel is purpura haemorrhagica* (see Chapter 13), which may occur during the immediate recovery phase, or during convalescence some 2 weeks later.

An early diagnosis in in-contact animals may be made by taking temperatures twice daily. At this early stage suitable antibiotic treatment may prevent any further development taking place, but it is usually considered dangerous to treat with antibiotics once abscesses have begun to form, as their development may be inhibited producing a phase of chronic abscessation, and a greater risk of complications occurring by bacteraemic spread.

Rhinitis (cold, nasal catarrh, or nasal gleet)

This is due to infection by one of several equine rhinoviruses. The syndrome has been known for many years, and was, in fact, common among young cart-horses. A slight clear bilateral nasal discharge is complicated by secondary bacteria and becomes profuse, mucopurulent and grey in colour. There is slight submandibular node enlargement and mild pharyngitis with occasional cough. The horse is only slightly unwell, and the temperature is usually normal. Nevertheless if the patient is worked, or stressed in other ways, the condition may become chronic and involve one or both sinuses with severe long-term results. A persistent mucopurulent nasal discharge, particularly if unilateral and foul smelling, should always cause suspicion of sinus involvement.

Equine influenza

A clinical syndrome caused by a group of myxoviruses. A considerable number are involved, but they fall into two main types.

A/Equi/1 was first isolated in Prague in 1956; then A/Equi 1/Cambridge 63: England 73: Pirbright 73: London 73, and so on. A/Equi/1 was the original influenza of this country, a mild condition known also as epizootic cough, stable cough, Newmarket cough, etc.

Then in 1965 *A/Equi 2/Miami/63* arrived from South America via the USA. 'American' flu was a much more severe clinical syndrome, and caused a nation-wide explosive outbreak.

Slowly over the years, however, widespread immunity developed, the clinical syndrome became less dramatic, and it is now very difficult to differentiate between A/Equi 1 and A/Equi 2 on clinical grounds alone. The main types still exist, but much drifting has occurred. New A/Equi 2 strains are Kentucky and Fontainbleu.

The clinical picture of influenza varies in severity according to the strain involved. Initially there is a high temperature (104°F (40°C) plus), with leucopenia and neutropenia. There are variable degrees of malaise, slightly enlarged submandibular lymph nodes, slight serous nasal discharge, lachrymation and a frequent cough. There is often laryngitis, and a varying degree of bronchitis. Enlargement of the subparotid lymph nodes sometimes occurs. Pressure on the larynx provokes the dry cough typical of the disease. By and large influenza is only dangerous in foals and aged horses, although complications may occur in any horse. Normally the horse feels better in 4 days, temperature should then be normal, but the cough persists for at least 2 weeks. Complete rest is all important. There must be good nursing and careful feeding during a long convalescence. The horse should not be worked for 4 weeks, or at least 2 weeks after all coughing has ceased. Neglect in this respect can lead to complications, e.g. pharyngitis, pharyngeal paralysis, conjunctivitis (pink eye), pneumonia, heart disease, purpura, ventral oedema and oedema of lower legs, laminitis, jaundice, enteritis, orchitis and abortion.

One must remember the long period of depression (postviral depression), which may follow influenza if the patient does not recieve a long enough rest. There is anaemia, leucopenia, neutropenia, with an increase in lymphocytes and (often) in monocytes. Many clinicians believe that a similar, but milder, depression may follow influenza vaccination unless the horse receives a period of rest of some fourteen days following the injection.

Equine influenza has been relatively rare in Britain in recent years, probably as a result of the widespread vaccination programme. A further explosive epidemic has, however, occurred in the summer and autumn of 1989. Suspicion of influenza may be confirmed by *virus isolation* from nasopharyngeal swabs taken early in the disease and sent to the laboratory in transport media, or by *serology*, using the haemagglutination inhibition test on paired samples taken in (1) the acute and (2) the convalescent phase.

Rhinopneumonitis (IVR: ERP)

This disease, nowadays called simply 'the cough' in racing circles, is caused by *equine herpes virus 1*. There are two subtypes – 1 and 2. Both produce respiratory signs, but those due to subtype 1 are very slight. Subtype 1 is much more important as a cause of abortion in the mare, and as a cause of paresis in horses reinfected by the virus after immunity due to previous infection has waned.

The respiratory form is most commonly seen in young horses but may occur at any age. The symptoms are comparatively mild. There is fever with temperature up to 106°F (41°C), with a slight cough, and large soft submandibular and parotid lymph nodes. Appetite is reduced and the nasal mucous membranes are congested. The temperature stays high for up to a week and is usually highest in the evening. There is considerable risk of secondary bacterial infection producing a persistent bronchitic cough and nasal discharge. Pneumonia is a possibility, and arteritis, taenosynovitis, bursitis, and oedema of the legs may also occur. These complications are much less likely to occur if the horse is rested completely for 4 weeks as soon as the disease appears. Antibiotics may also help. Immunity is very short, only 4–6 months, and reinfection may produce lethargy and poor performance without obvious respiratory signs. Confirmation of diagnosis again depends on the isolation of EHV 1 from nasal swabs collected in transport media, and serology from paired samples. Differential diagnosis obviously includes influenza, but there is much less coughing, less nasal discharge, and considerably more swelling of submandibular and parotid lymph nodes. These may be sufficiently enlarged to lead to an erroneous diagnosis of strangles, but they do not fluctuate, nor rupture, and eventually subside again.

Other viruses possibly occurring in respiratory conditions of horses

(1) *Equine herpes virus 2* – a slow-growing virus which occurs in unweaned foals causing coughing, profuse nasal mucus and 'scalding' of the nostrils; adults may show poor performance and profuse nasal discharge, plus a slight cough.
(2) *Adenovirus* produces a fatal respiratory disease in Arab foals suffering from combined immunodeficiency. Adenovirus also causes a fairly vague respiratory disease in young horses, which may develop soft faeces.
(3) *Reovirus* has caused respiratory infections on the continent.

Diagnostic techniques applicable to all the respiratory viruses include the use of nasopharyngeal swabs placed in transport media and sent, chilled, to the laboratory. These viruses may be cultured on egg amnion, or kidney from foals, rabbits or horses.

Serological tests are also useful. They include:

(1) Haemagglutination and haemagglutination inhibition tests for influenza viruses.
(2) Plaque reduction tests for herpes and rhinoviruses.
(3) Agar gel precipitation tests for adenoviruses.

The Animal Health Trust's Virology Unit is at Lanwades Park, Kennett, Newmarket, Suffolk CB8 7PN.

Chronic pulmonary disease (CPD)

This is also known as chronic allergic obstructive expiratory disease (CAOED). If one is presented with a horse perfectly well in itself, with normal temperature and pulse rate, housed, with access to hay or straw, with an abnormal respiratory pattern with an abdominal component, and an occasional cough or group of coughs, then almost beyond doubt it is suffering from this disease, which is, of course, allergic in nature. The allergens include many moulds of the micropolyspora group, particularly *Mycobacterium faeni*, which is involved in human 'farmer's lung'. *Aspergillus* spp. may also be involved, and the condition is exacerbated by the dust and debris so often associated with mouldy hay.

Allergy may develop insidiously, so that the owner is unable to pinpoint accurately the onset of the disease. In other cases it may be present in a latent form from very early life, and is then triggered off by a respiratory infection, usually of virus origin. This is important clinically for it explains the common history that all was well until the horse caught 'flu and then the chronic cough developed so it must be a complication of 'flu, e.g. bronchitis. Alternatively, one is told that all the horses in the stable developed 'the cough' but that this one has never recovered.

Rarely the disease starts as acute allergic pulmonary disease which looks exactly like an acute asthmatic attack in the human, and then tails off into the usual chronic form. This acute asthmatic form usually occurs when a horse which has been at grass since last winter is for some reason suddenly housed, if only for half an hour or so. The attack develops almost explosively. The attendant is frequently alerted by the very loud respiratory, particularly expiratory sounds which may be heard from many yards away. There is swinging abdominal breathing with a spectacular 'double lift' or 'heave'; the mouth is often a little open with foam about the lips; coughing is loud and paroxysmal in nature; pulse may be between 70 and 80 per minute; temperature slightly raised due to the tremendous exertion, and sweating may be profuse. The horse stands with 'a leg at each corner' and its head held low. Lung sounds are loud, harsh, and greatly exaggerated. Nostils are flared. Steroidal and non-steroidal anti-inflammatory drugs, e.g. corticosteroids and flunixin (Finadyne) may be used and their effect may be to all intents and purposes diagnostic, for within half an hour to an hour, particularly if the animal is returned to grass, it is likely to be to all intents and purposes normal, although from this point onwards the chronic disease may be noticed.

The chronic disease (CPD) is linked with modern hay making and baling techniques. Humidity in the bale tends to be high, and moulds develop well in such an environment. There is a marked variation from horse to horse in their tendency to become allergic. Nevertheless many experienced clinicians in horse and pony practice believe that practically every housed horse is showing some degree of CPD by the end of each winter. It is only a slight exaggeration to say that if one looks at a stabled horse at rest and *notices* that it is breathing, then that horse has CPD. Bronchiolar spasm accentuated by bronchiolitis, resulting from the allergic reaction plus dust and debris, cause narrowing of the airways, obstruction and irritation. The coughing leads to dilation and overinflation of the lungs, which means that they will not empty completely by their own elasticity, but require the abdominal push or 'heave' so characteristic of the disease, and known as the 'double lift'. Originally it was believed that emphysema was a characteristic part of the condition, but in fact the condition is one of pulmonary overinflation, not pulmonary emphysema, until eventually in neglected cases degrees of irreversible emphysema may supervene. There may, therefore, be little or no abnormal lung sound, although it is often possible to map out the extended borders of the area of auscultation and percussion due to overinflation. This lack of emphysematous sound may be confusing to clinicians who have been brought up to expect it.

Once emphysema has occurred the next stage, now largely historical, is circulatory obstruction in the lung eventually producing right heart dilatation.

Nevertheless the majority of cases seen today are relatively mild. There is an occasional soft non-productive cough, or series of coughs, sounding more like clearing of the throat. Coughing is more noticeable at night; when the horse is brought out into the cold morning air; and particularly when it starts to trot. There may be an occasional retching sound before the cough ('he's got something stuck in his throat'). Sometimes the cough develops later in the disease when the respiratory pattern is already obvious. It is worth trying to elicit the characteristic cough by squeezing the first or second tracheal ring *gently*, but this does not always work, and may in any case cause coughing in other respiratory diseases. The respiratory pattern develops slowly and may not be obvious at first. It is essential to wait until the horse settles and stands still. Watch the flank obliquely and in good light, preferably sunlight. Inspiration is normal: the first expiratory phase is a quick relaxation of the rib cage which the observer may miss if not concentrating. The second phase is a long smooth push involving muscles of the flank. There is not necessarily a definite pause between phases. Watch the anus – it protrudes with the second phase. Listen with a stethoscope over the trachea – the two phases can be distinctly heard. Place your ear or cheek close to the horse's nostril – the two phases are clearly felt in its breath on your face. The first is a quick puff, the second long drawn out and slowly dying away. Usually the only abnormal lung sound is a bronchitic sound in the anterior part of the middle third of the chest, i.e. over the tracheal bifurcation. If emphysema finally develops it will be along the ventral and posterior lung edges of the diaphragmatic lobes. The sound can be likened to the clicking of many knitting needles, or the sound of granulated sugar being shaken on brown paper. It is best heard during the second expiratory phase when the emphysematous edges of the diaphragmatic lobes are under pressure.

There is sometimes a mucopurulent nasal discharge which can get quite profuse – this is due to the bronchitic part of the syndrome. It is well worth while shaking up a hay sample under the patient's nose – positive cases are likely to cough. In the racehorse living by and large in better ventilated boxes under more enlightened management, the respiratory pattern and cough are less obvious, but the mucopurulent discharge more so. There is much congestion of the mucous membrane at the bronchial tree, and, under the stress of racing, haemorrhage may occur here and appear as spots of blood in the discharge, most noticeable when the horse rests after racing and lowers his head to eat or drink. The syndrome is known as exercise-induced pulmonary haemorrhage (EIPH). The fluid which accumulates in the pharynx while galloping tends to be excessive and occasionally seems to cause choking in racehorses suffering from CPD.

Pollen allergy

Very occasionally during hot dry spells in mid summer an allergy to certain grass pollens, e.g. ryegrass, may be seen. Symptoms include a serous nasal discharge, lachrymation and cough.

Parasitic bronchitis (lungworm disease)

This may be seen during late summer and autumn in horses which have been in contact with donkeys and are infested by *Dictyocaulus arnfeldi*, the donkey lungworm. The horse is not a natural host and infection tends not to become patent. Larvae are seldom found in the faeces, making definitive diagnosis difficult; but this does mean that horse seldom infects horse, so there is usually a donkey somewhere in the relatively recent environment, if one is aware of the probability and takes time to look. Affected horses may lose some condition and do not look as well as the average CPD sufferer. Coughing is more forceful and tends to be paroxysmal. The head is held low and there is saliva at the lips after each paroxysm of coughing. A double expiratory movement is not characteristic of this disease, and lung sounds are much more apparent with moist rales and moist bronchitic sounds, but emphysema is seldom present. Most horses affected by lungworm have recovered by late winter at the latest, but the occasional patient does not seem to develop resistance and may become heavily infested and quite seriously ill, with extreme pneumonic lesions. Differential diagnosis between parasitic bronchitis and CPD may be difficult in the autumn in horses which are out at grass by day and housed at night. A practical differentiation may be made by treating with a wide-spectrum anthelmintic such as oxfenbendazole or ivermectin and then housing for a fortnight or so. The lungworm case almost invariably improves markedly, but the CPD case gets worse until it is returned to grass again.

Nasopharyngeal lymphoid hyperplasia

Universal in young horses. The condition consists of small diffusely arranged nodular lymphoid swellings all over the nasopharyngeal mucosa, giving a studded effect. These swellings are seen first in many young foals, and enlarge as the growing horse meets viral antigens. They disappear by middle age, but get bigger and appear inflamed during infections. It is now believed that the condition is not a disease picture, but a normal defensive mechanism.

9 Respiratory disease – the dyspnoeic horse

Diaphragmatic hernia
Pleurisy, pleural effusion, transit fever
Pneumonia
Thoracic lymphosarcoma
Other thoracic neoplasms
Marie's disease
Tuberculosis
Acute anaphylactic shock
Acute venous congestion of lungs

Diaphragmatic hernia

This can cause considerable diagnostic difficulty. Fortunately it occurs very rarely, but should always be considered in horses showing colic and/or dyspnoea which have recent or healed wounds of the thorax, or which have a history of recent thoracic trauma.

Three main clinical forms occur but there may be considerable overlapping of diagnostic signs:

(1) Congenital diaphragmatic defects do occur, and may not lead to clinical signs until the animal is well grown. The hernial aperture is usually small and the prolapsed material is generally no more than a short loop of small intestine and some omentum. There are unlikely to be any respiratory signs and abdominal pain from the incarcerated gut is generally slight and very difficult to locate. The whole lesion may be small and difficult to find even during abdominal surgery.

(2) Traumatic diaphragmatic hernia may occur, resulting in the incarceration or strangulation of the small intestine. Helpful signs of chest injury are not always present, and it is very easy to diagnose an acute small intestine condition without realizing that a hernia is involved. If there is any suspicion of respiratory abnormality careful auscultation and percussion of the chest must be carried out. It must be remembered, however, that there are often quite loud borborygmi in the normal chest, arising from the oesophagus, while on the other hand there may be changes in the respiratory pattern of the normal chest in colic cases arising from metabolic change.

(3) Whilst herniation of the small intestine does not usually interfere unduly with the respiratory pattern and behaves much more like a gut obstruction, the large intestine may become involved in the hernia. This is much more bulky than the small gut and causes very serious swinging dyspnoea, but does not cause the same degree of gut pain – large gut involvement is rarely, if ever, as painful as small. If there is absence or near absence of lung sounds, usually much more marked on one side of the chest; if percussion produces a dull sound over this same area; if gut sounds can be heard over the same area; and if thoracocentesis produces fluid, then you are reasonably certain of yourself. Rectal examination revealing a surprisingly empty abdomen helps to confirm the diagnosis.

It is worth remembering that surgical repair is very difficult: not only is the site relatively inaccessible, but it is practically impossible to maintain normal intrathoracic pressure during the course of the operation.

Pleurisy, pleural effusion, 'transit fever', stress

Most equine pleurisy is stress related, often associated with periods of severe fatigue. In recent years it has been associated with long journeys, particularly by air. If the journey is long with several stops the condition may appear while the horse is still in transit. Otherwise it shows clinically from 4 to 14 days after reaching the destination. The usual organisms are *Streptococcus zooepidemicus*, *Streptococcus equi* and *Pasteurella* spp., all of which are found as commensal organisms in the equine environment.

The clinical picture is severe. The patient is much depressed, with pyrexia (temperature: 104–105°F, 40–40.5°C) which slowly disappears as the disease progresses. Pulse rate is also high, and may be up to 100 per minute. If the temperature falls while the pulse rate remains high, the prognosis is grave. There is often sweating, and considerable pain which can easily be confused with abdominal pain, but, in fact, represents dry pleurisy. There is occasional painful coughing, and an obvious pleuritic line. The chest rapidly fills with a profuse straw-coloured and often frothy inflammatory exudate. When sufficient has formed the respiratory pain ceases and the respiratory pattern becomes swinging and laboured. At this stage there may be at least 30 litres of fluid in the chest. The pulse, although still fast, becomes much weaker. There may be some pulmonary involvement. The fluid level may be detected by auscultation or radiography.

Drainage using a wide-bore needle with a two-way tap and drainage tube can be carried out via the seventh intercostal space just in front of the eighth rib (to avoid the intercostal vessels). Local anaesthetic and aseptic precautions should be used.

Pneumonia

Pneumonia is rare as a primary entity in the horse, but fatigue, cold and stress can predispose and the horse succumbs to its own commensal organisms. Temperature is 103–105°F

(39.5–40.5°C). Pulse is weak and rapid. The horse looks very ill with head held low. Marked dyspnoea, occasional cough, and a variety of rales and bronchial sounds are present. Inhalation pneumonia can occur after drenching or stomach tubing. There may be moist rales from the ventral aspects of the lungs. Gangrenous lesions develop and the gangrene smell may be detected on the horse's breath. Temperature tends to remain relatively low (102°F, 39°C) and then become subnormal whilst pulse rate becomes faster and weaker. Prognosis is always grave.

Occasionally a twig or similar object gets into the trachea and sticks at the tracheal bifurcation – confirmation is by endoscope.

Thoracic (mediastinal) lymphosarcoma

Lymphosarcomatous disease produces several relatively distinct syndromes in the horse, although a certain amount of overlapping may occur. The thoracic form shows a fairly rapid onset, with oedema around the thoracic inlet and back along the ventral thorax. Sometimes oedema affects the ventral abdomen as well, and even the legs. Weight loss is rapid. There is often a palpable mass, consisting of hyperplastic lymphoid tissue, on one or both sides of the neck in the jugular furrow at the thoracic inlet. Pyrexia, either continuous or intermittent, is usually present. Dyspnoea develops slowly, and may become severe, with marked swinging abdominal movement and elbows abducted. Dysphagia may be present due to pressure of lymphosarcomatous masses, and causes saliva to be returned to the mouth and dribbled. There may be a cough. Auscultation and radiography reveal a fluid line, and some 20 litres of a blood-tinged, frothy, modified transudate, containing lymphoblasts and lymphoid cells, may be removed by thoracic paracentesis. The pulse rate is raised, often markedly. Distension of the jugular veins is a noticeable and regular feature. Euthanasia is usually necessary in little more than a week. Haematology may show leucopenia, but leucocytosis and neutrophilia are more likely. There is no lymphocytosis. There may be a secondary hyperlipaemia.

Post-mortem examination shows a massive intrathoracic effusion. Parts of the ventral lobes of the lungs may be collapsed. There are lymphosarcomatous masses in the anterior mediastinum. These are not thymic in origin: they result from the coalescence of hugely enlarged lymphatic nodes. Other thoracic lymph nodes may also be involved, as may some abdominal nodes.

Other types of thoracic neoplasia

These are occasionally seen, e.g. carcinoma.

Marie's disease (pulmonary hypertrophic osteoarthropathy)

A rare condition usually seen in dogs, but which does occur in horses. Masses in the chest, usually neoplastic, in some way trigger off painful bony swellings on the bones of the lower limbs.

Tuberculosis

Avian tuberculosis still occurs in horses. The sources are fowls and pheasants. Lesions occur in the equine liver, spleen and lymph nodes producing granulomatous masses and weight loss, and in the colon producing a Johne's-like picture.

Bovine tuberculosis is now very rare in cattle and extinct in horses. But the recent increase in the bovine incidence may mean that the occasional case will occur in the horse. The lesions are chronic proliferative granulomatous tumour-like masses in the liver, spleen and lymph nodes. Lesions are also seen affecting the cervical vertebrae and causing a stiff neck; a similar picture to that occurring in brucellosis, and in vertebral trauma. There is much weight loss. The terminal phase, however, may be miliary tuberculosis of the lungs, giving an apparently pneumonic picture in an emaciated horse.

Acute anaphylactic shock

This condition may well have a very sudden onset. Within minutes the horse becomes cold to the touch, clammy, and wet with sweat. It shivers, is obviously anxious, and shows very shallow rapid respirations. Temperature is often subnormal, but pulse rate very fast, often over 100 per minute. Considerable numbers of oedematous plaques may appear over much of the body surface.

Acute venous congestion of the lungs

A condition sometimes seen in an unfit horse pushed too hard at too fast a pace. There is severe pulmonary congestion, with blood-flecked froth at the nostrils, profuse sweating, a raised temperature, and a fast wildly beating heart. The horse pulls up in severe distress and may even collapse. It is vital that no attempt be made to move the animal. If it is allowed complete rest it will probably soon be normal again, although no attempt should be made to work it for several weeks.

Conditions simulating dyspnoea

Diseases producing exaggerated respiratory movement from causes other than respiratory embarrassment can easily be misdiagnosed as respiratory tract disease. Any condition producing exaggerated respiratory movement will produce harsh lung sounds which may easily be misdiagnosed as true pulmonary or bronchitic sounds:

(1) *Hypocalcaemia* – see Chapter 20.
(2) *Transit tetany* – see Chapter 20.
(3) *Synchronous diaphragmatic flutter* – see Chapter 20.
(4) *Heatstroke* – see Chapter 20.

10 Dysphagia – difficulty in swallowing

Mouth, lips, teeth
Cranial nerve damage (fifth or seventh)
Tetanus
Thoracic lymphosarcoma
Lead poisoning
Hyperlipaemia
Polymyositis
Botulism
Guttural pouch
Pharyngitis
Pharyngeal nerve paralysis
'Choke'
Grass disease

This is a relatively common syndrome in the horse and presents wide and varied diagnostic possibilities.

Mouth, lips, teeth

If a horse has any difficulty in taking food and water into its mouth, chewing food, and passing it into the oropharynx preparatory to swallowing it, a full examination of the mouth should be made for *cuts and ulcers on the tongue and lips, obvious dental abnormalities, and foreign bodies in the mouth*, e.g. the crown of a temporary molar remaining fixed on the crown of the permanent tooth after eruption. In such cases there may be mouth discomfort and salivation, but the horse is not ill, and apart from its mouth will seem quite normal.

Cranial nerve damage

Paralysis of the facial (seventh cranial) nerve slackens the affected cheek and lip, and the loss of tone in the affected muscles causes the muzzle to be pulled towards the normal side. Food and water drop from the mouth on the affected side. If the condition is bilateral there is no such deviation and the whole muzzle looks slack. In such cases drinking may be particularly difficult unless the horse plunges its muzzle deeply into the water so that the commissures of the lips are covered. In most cases the nerve has been affected by an injury to the side of the face or head, but if nerve damage is central the ear and the upper eyelid on the affected side may lack tone – the ear may droop and the upper eyelid slacken, neither shutting nor opening completely. Occasionally, the fifth nerve may be affected, in which case the horse cannot quite close its mouth, so that water and saliva dribble from the mouth intermittently. This can be checked by lifting the lower jaw quickly when the upper and lower teeth will be heard to click together.,

Tetanus

Tetanus interferes with prehension as a result of muscle spasm causing trismus. The horse cannot eat nor drink. Diagnosis should present no difficulty, for the generalized muscle spasm and exaggerated response to stimuli typical of the disease follow trismus very rapidly. The membrana nictitans is in spasm across the eye.

Thoracic lymphosarcoma

The passage of saliva down the oesophagus is obstructed by the lymphosarcomatous mass in the mediastinum and at the entrance to the chest. Saliva collects in the mouth, and the horse smacks its lips upon the accumulating liquid. (See Chapter 3.)

Lead poisoning

Excessive salivation and varying degrees of pharyngeal paralysis are seen in lead poisoning. Saliva and water may come down the nose and drip from the mouth. Laryngeal paralysis may cause a loud laryngeal 'roaring'. The horse may be dull, wandering aimlessly, with defective vision. Diagnosis depends on blood-lead levels in life, and at post-mortem on liver and kidney levels.

Hyperlipaemia (see Chapter 6)

This is associated with a maxillary myositis which interferes with prehension of food and water. The pony may stand over the water bucket attempting to drink, but succeeds only in splashing. As in most conditions preventing a horse from drinking, the frenzied attempts to drink may spill most of the contents of the bucket on to the floor, suggesting to the groom that the water has been drunk. It is essential to wait and watch after offering the horse water.   ·

Polymyositis (muscular dystrophy)

Much more generalized muscular lesions are seen – the pony salivates but cannot swallow its saliva. Nor can it swallow water which returns down the nose. All muscles are stiff and painful, pulse rate very high, gait stilted and staggering, respiration shallow and fast, with sweating and marked distress. Eventually recumbency occurs, soon followed by death. The oesophagus is often found with much food material in it; the muscular lesions involve the oesophagus and other involuntary muscle as well. Creatine phosphokinase (CPK) and aspartate aminotransferse (AST) are very high.

Botulism

Botulism causes weakness and progressive paralysis of all muscle. The horse becomes slowly weak, stumbles, and lies down, first in sternal and then in lateral recumbency. It remains peaceful and apparently relaxed with a minimum of weak leg movement. It cannot eat, finds difficulty in drinking, and much water runs down the nose. Both prehension and swallowing are affected. Occasional very mild cases occur in which the horse can walk in a somewhat slow relaxed manner, but cannot drink, and has to be kept hydrated by stomach tube until able to drink for itself. Definitive diagnosis of botulism is by isolating the toxin at post-mortem. This requires specialized laboratory facilities.

Guttural pouch

Guttural pouch diphtheresis does not interfere with swallowing, but guttural pouch empyema may occasionally do so if the pouch is very distended, particularly if the condition is bilateral, and even more so if there are large concretions in one or both pouches. The distension is noticeable in Viborg's triangle and behind the vertical ramus. Confirmation of diagnosis is by endoscopy, or lateral radiography.

Guttural pouch tympany in the foal, however, is much more likely to cause dysphagia. The tympany, especially if bilateral, may be sufficient to cause dysphagia with milk running back down the nose, and even some obstructive pressure on the trachea. The other cause of dysphagia in the foal is cleft palate, which, from birth, involves difficulty in swallowing because milk easily passes into the nasal chambers and runs down the nose, or even, sometimes, down the trachea.

Pharyngitis

Pharyngitis may occur, often as a complication of influenza. Some cases may be quite severe with a raised temperature and pulse rate, and considerable painful inflammatory swelling and oedema of the pharyngeal mucous membrane. The condition is known to the layman as 'quinzy', and causes both pain and difficulty in swallowing. As so often in dysphagia it is much easier to swallow food than water, and much of the water comes down the nose.

Paralysis of the pharyngeal nerves

A sequel to upper respiratory tract virus infections, and not uncommon after equine influenza epidemics. Symptoms usually appear some 2–3 weeks after the virus infection – swallowing may be practically impossible and both food and water are returned down the nose causing emaciation and dehydration in a very short time. On the other hand the condition may be slight and even unnoticed – there is a little difficulty in drinking and drops of water may appear at the nostrils. Grass is the food most easily swallowed, but a green stain appears at the nostrils. Pharyngeal nerve paralysis may sometimes be associated with guttural pouch infection.

'Choke'

Choke is a frequent cause of dysphagia in the horse. It occasionally occurs where the oesophagus passes the heart, and occasionally at the diaphragm, but the usual site involves the first 6 inches (15 cm) or so of the oesophagus. In the past, bran was the common offending material, but in recent years choke has usually been due to sugar beet pulp or sugar beet nuts fed without proper soaking. The horse is obviously uncomfortable; it arches its neck and makes swallowing movements. Water and debris are usually noticeable at the nostrils; attempts to drink cause discomfort and choking; there may be coughing. The impaction can often be felt in the oesophageal groove on the left side of the neck. After the impacted food has moved, symptoms may not disappear for a day or two because the oesophagus will be oedematous and sore and will still constitute an uncomfortable obstruction.

Grass disease

In many areas of this country this is the most important cause of dysphagia. Acute grass disease is not usually difficult to diagnose: the horse is obviously uncomfortable; swallowing is impossible; a sticky mixture of food and water is often seen at the nostrils. There may be eructation and forceful painful regurgitation of greenish fluid stomach content via the nose. Pulse rate is raised, but temperature is in normal range. No faeces are passed. There is abdominal discomfort, patchy sweating around the tail base, behind the elbows and in front of the stifles. Muscular tremors are evident particularly over the flanks. The clinical picture is dramatic. The chronic form is much more confusing. The picture here is primarily loss of condition over many days or even weeks. The horse is tucked up and herring gutted with back arched and the tail clamped down.

There is a tendency to stand with all four feet close together and the head and neck stretched forward. The penis is relaxed; there is muscle tremor and patchy sweating. Practically no faeces are passed; rarely there is scanty cow-like diarrhoea. Chronic cases will eat little, preferably grass, but have great difficulty in swallowing. It is even more difficult to drink; water and green stains come down the nose. There is often abdominal discomfort after eating or drinking. There is haemoconcentration, and PCV (packed cell volume) is often raised. Total serum protein is often raised and blood urea is always high.

11 Nasal discharge

Upper respiratory tract infections
  Strangles
  Influenza
  Rhinopneumonitis
  Rhinitis
Chronic pulmonary disease
Guttural pouch disease
Sinusitis
Conditions of the nasal chambers
  Necrosis of the turbinates
  Neoplastic lesions of the nasal chambers,
    e.g. ethnoid haematoma
All causes of dysphagia

Nasal discharge in the horse is a common state of affairs. The aetiological factors include:

Upper respiratory tract infections

(1) *Strangles* – serous discharge which becomes purulent and profuse.
(2) *Virus infections:*
    (a) *Influenza.*
    (b) *Rhinopneumonitis.*
        Influenza causes more nasal discharge than rhino-pneumonitis, and often causes lachrymal discharge as well.
    (c) *Rhinitis* where the discharge may become profuse, mucopurulent and chronic.

Chronic pulmonary disease

This disease is characterized by a chronic cough and biphasic expiratory movements. Nasal discharge is variable, and when present may be mucoid or mucopurulent. In horses with chronic pulmonary disease working at fast paces there may be a mucoid discharge with small quantities of blood floating on it, which appears when the horse pulls up after galloping and puts its head down to eat or drink.

Guttural pouch disease

When guttural pouch empyema occurs it is *likely* to be unilateral, and the fairly profuse pus formed is discharged largely through the nostril on the affected side. Diagnosis is aided by catheterization, endoscopy or lateral radiography, and is easier if a chondroid concretion is present. Guttural pouch diphtheresis is also *likely* to be unilateral, but does not produce pus. There may, however, be episodes of haemorrhage, and there is often a definite necrotic smell at the relevant nostril, particularly when the condition has been present for some time and there is damage to the neighbouring tissues by extension of the invading fungal organisms. Haemorrhage may be quite severe, and even dangerous. Diagnosis is by endoscopy, looking for blood leaking from the Eustachian tube, or for fungal patches overlying the internal carotid artery. Sometimes the external carotid artery is affected.

Sinuses

Acute sinus infection may occur producing mucopurulent nasal discharge, usually from one nostril, i.e. unilateral. Much more serious is chronic sinusitis with persistent mucopurulent nasal discharge, again usually unilateral, and the result of an acute upper respiratory tract infection. Eventually a necrotic smell develops, and in longstanding cases there may even be facial swelling. This is particularly likely to happen if, as sometimes occurs, the cause of the sinusitis is infection of the roots of the last three molar teeth. Lateral radiography of the maxillary sinus may help the diagnosis.

Nasal chambers

(1) *Necrosis of the turbinate bones* occasionally occurs.
(2) *Neoplastic lesions* of the nasal chambers are also sometimes seen. *Ethnoid haematomas* are among such lesions. This tumour is vascular in nature containing a massive blood clot, and is another possible reason for serious unilateral nasal haemorrhage. Confirmation of diagnosis is by endoscopy or lateral radiography.

Dysphagia

The differential diagnosis of conditions interfering with prehension or with swallowing has already been considered. The conditions interfering with swallowing itself are also among the causes of nasal discharge, the nasal discharge being a mixture of food, grass, water and saliva in varying proportions.

12 Salivation

Lead poisoning
Organophosphorus poisoning
Rhododendron poisoning
Injuries and foreign bodies in the mouth

Salivation will obviously be clinically noticeable to a greater or lesser extent in most of the conditions already described in Chapter 10 on difficulty in prehension, and dysphagia, for if saliva cannot be swallowed it accumulates in the mouth or oropharynx and either leaks between the lips or appears down the nostrils.

In some conditions, however, saliva may be formed in excess and becomes an embarrassment for this reason.

(1) *Lead poisoning* which causes direct stimulation of the salivary centre (see Chapter 10).

(2) *Organophosphorus poisoning* which causes excessive salivation, increased tear production, scanty diarrhoea, patchy sweating, tremors and varying abdominal pain.

(3) *Rhododendron poisoning* which involves excess salivation, vomiting and varying degrees of diarrhoea.

(4) *Injuries in the mouth,* particularly foreign bodies wedged between the teeth, etc.

13 Allergic and anaphylactic conditions

Acute anaphylactic shock
Purpura haemorrhagica
Urticaria and skin allergies
Sweet-itch (mane and tail eczema)
Chronic pulmonary disease
Head flicking

It has been said that 'the horse is a histaminic and oedematous animal'. It is certainly true that the veterinary surgeon attends allergic or anaphylactic syndromes relatively frequently.

Acute anaphylactic shock

This has already been described in Chapter 9. Notice that numbers of oedematous plaques develop over much of the body during the recovery period. They vary in diameter from half an inch to several inches and disappear within 24–36 hours. Some cases were associated with warble fly larvae.

Purpura haemorrhagica

This is believed to represent an anaphylactic reaction to *Streptococcus equi* infection. It tends to follow strangles, streptococcal wound infection, and the streptococcal complications of virus infections, usually appearing about a fortnight after recovery has taken place. Sometimes there has not been any obvious, i.e. clinical, primary infection. The first signs are usually oedema of the nostrils followed by oedema over the whole head, which may be sufficiently extensive to interfere with the airway, producing respiratory embarrassment. Some degree of dysphagia may also occur. Then oedema of the limbs develops, usually more severe in the hind limbs. The oedematous areas are abruptly demarcated near the elbows and stifles giving the effect known as 'bottle-limb'. There are often plaques of oedema from 1 to 5 inches (2.5–12.5 cm) in diameter elsewhere on the body. All the oedematous areas are cool and painless, and begin to exude serum which forms crusts on the skin. The oedematous areas are very prone to pressure necrosis, so that great care is needed with clothing, etc. Plaques may disappear while others appear. Damage to capillary vessels occurs with leakage of blood into the tissues. Petechial haemorrhages are seen on the nasal mucous membranes; the conjunctival membranes, where blood-stained tears may occur; inside the lips; and on the tongue. These haemorrhages are sometimes ecchymoses rather than petechiae. Anaemia develops. There is leucocytosis and neutrophilia with a left shift. Blood calcium falls. Body temperature seldom rises significantly, but there is a rapid pulse. Any marked temperature rise indicates secondary infection and is a poor prognostic sign. There is often oedema of the lungs with exudation producing fluid sounds, and marked dyspnoea. Considerable serous exudation may discharge through the nostrils. The gut may also be affected, with oedema, haemorrhage and necrosis, causing colic and blood-stained diarrhoea. This is also prognostically grave. Mortality in acute cases may easily be 50% but many milder cases occur. In fact a wide gradation of severity occurs from mild oedema and respiratory embarrassment on the one hand to the acute picture described above on the other.

Urticaria and skin allergies

Various manifestations of oedematous development may occur without any suggestion that the horse is feeling unwell – one may find large numbers of tiny oedematous papules no more than 0.25 inches (0.65 cm) in diameter covering much of the shoulders, neck, chest and even flanks. This manifestation is often spoken of among the horse fraternity as 'humour' and generally appears in fit animals with a very high concentrate food intake.

Urticarial lesions vary in size from 0.25 inches (0.65 cm) diameter to large plaques, and even to extensive ventral oedema which has to be differentiated from the oedema associated with albumin loss through gut or kidney, and failure to produce albumin by the liver. The urticarial case, however, does not feel ill apart from pruritis in some cases, and some respiratory embarrassment if any pulmonary oedema is present. In most cases recovery is rapid and spontaneous, although steroid and possibly antihistamine treatment may accelerate resolution. Occasionally in cases showing pruritis, rubbing and biting, the skin may become infected, delaying healing. Suggested causes for urticaria include food, saddle soap, drugs, bacteria, nettles, gnats, flies, mosquitoes, warbles and heel mites. Many of the larger plaques along neck, chest and flank are believed to be due to biting flies, while oedema of the conjunctiva and the eyelids on fly-infested summer days may well be due to flies which often almost hide the nasal canthus from view, and cause dermatitis and ulceration of the skin at this site plus excessive lachrymation. It has been suggested that the extensive ventral oedema which is seen occasionally in summer on rich pastures may be due to allergic reaction to proteins in grass juices entering the system via grazes on the ventral abdomen when the horse is recumbent. There is, however, very little conclusive evidence for this possibility. Nevertheless it does seem probable that the oozing eczematous lesions seen occasionally on the muzzle and coronets of horses grazing on summer pasture with some clover content may be due to a contact allergy.

Sweet-itch (mane and tail eczema)

Sweet-itch is caused by allergy to culicoides midges. The disease is also said to have a familial incidence, and it is interesting that, for whatever reason, foals of affected dams not infrequently become affected themselves. The allergic reaction sets up pruritic areas of self-inflicted 'wet eczema' along both sides of the crest, and at the tail head. There may be much hair loss from the mane and tail. Lesions of various sizes may appear at the withers, along the back and over the quarters, but these are not always present. During the winter, lesions heal leaving hairless areas of thickened skin, which are usually covered again with new hair before the condition reappears in the following spring.

Chronic pulmonary disease

See Chapter 8.

Head flicking

See Chapter 20.

14 Muscular problems

The 'tied-up' syndrome
Azoturia
Polymyositis (muscular dystrophy)

The horse presents a considerable variety of muscle lesions, the aetiology of which is still very vague, previous traditional ideas being regarded as highly dubious. For convenience, and to avoid producing further aetiological confusion, it has now become usual to consider all the non-traumatic muscle conditions under the general heading of *equine rhabdomyolysis*. This includes:

The 'tied-up' syndrome ('cramped' or 'setfast')

This is usually seen in riding horses, e.g. hunters, eventers and steeplechasers. It occurs without any obvious common aetiological factor apart from a good level of food intake and bodily condition, and the fact that the clinical picture occurs during exercise. It may be no more than slight stiffness and shortened stride. More severe cases pull up, and may even exhibit slight myoglobinuria. Normally very rapid recovery occurs during rest periods, but the tendency towards recurrence is high.

Azoturia

This condition, also known as paralytic myoglobinuria, is much more severe. It usually, but by no means always, occurs in horses in good bodily condition, but with irregular exercise patterns, so that fairly severe exercise can follow several days' rest on full feed, which traditionally, but by no means always factually, is high in energy. It does not occur after one day's rest on full feed, but after several such quiet days. This typical food/exercise pattern, however, may be very variable. The symptoms appear some 10–15 minutes after fast work – even trotting – begins. The horse begins to sweat and respirations become fast and exaggerated. The gait is often described as rolling, but in most cases 'sinking' would be a better description. Stifles, fetlocks and hocks gradually become more and more flexed as the horse moves along until it can no longer support itself, and it collapses. It cannot rise onto its hindquarters. The gluteal and lumbar muscles particularly feel hard and swollen, and are painful on pressure. Urination is difficult, and the urine varies from dark brown to black depending on the severity of the case, and the degree of myoglobinuria. Occasionally the pectoral muscles are affected, in which case the forelimb will not bear weight and straddles sideways. Horses which have suffered an attack of azoturia seem to be prone to further attacks, and eventually survivors develop fibrosis and atrophy of the affected lumbar and gluteal muscles. Although it is convenient to consider the 'tied-up' syndrome and azoturia separately, nowadays one sees a gradation in clinical severity from the mildest 'tied-up' cases to the most severe azoturia cases, making it difficult to separate them into different categories. All cases in the range will show elevated creatine phosphokinase (CPK) and aspartate aminotransferase (AST) levels, the CPK levels rising to 50 000 iu/l plus, and the AST to 2000 iu/l plus in the worst azoturia cases.

Polymyositis (muscular dystrophy)

This condition has been seen for some 30 years but has only recently been widely recognized. It is a spectacular syndrome seen most frequently in undernourished ponies in marginal areas. The suggestion has been made, but never proven, that it is associated with a low selenium/vitamin E status in these ponies. Figures for selenium as low as half the accepted normals for the horse have been recorded in these cases, but normal ponies in the same group may also show very low figures. Sudden unaccustomed exercise may precipitate the clinical picture, e.g. mixing with a new group of ponies or putting on to a very large fresh pasture.

First signs may be mild colicky pain, some sweating, and scanty dark faeces (often mistaken for colic). The pony becomes dull, lying down more than usual, stiff legged (differential diagnosis tetanus), cannot get its head down to grass, straddles legs, or grazes on knees. Uncomfortable grunting occurs. It is particularly stiff over shoulders and forelegs; getting slowly worse, it can only drink if the bucket is held up to its head. Drinking gets difficult; it splashes in water without taking it in. It becomes difficult for the pony to rise from the recumbent position. Faeces are still passed. After a few hours the pony becomes distressed; respirations are rapid; it gets up and down; chewed grass and saliva stays in its mouth or comes down its nose. More sweating occurs. Pulse rate is now 80 plus a minute, but temperature does not rise. The urine becomes dark and contains myoglobin. The pony adopts a trestle attitude, i.e. 'a leg at each corner'. The head is held low, membranes become injected, faeces cease to pass, the bladder becomes very full; passage of a stomach tube shows that the pharynx and oesophagus are impacted with saliva-sodden grass. Choking sounds occur. Jaundice may be noticeable. In another hour or so the pony is in full lateral recumbency, agitated, apprehensive and struggling to rise. Respirations are now fast, jerky and abdominal, the nostrils dilated. Soon the pony is ploughing in a circle, very distressed, and euthanasia is essential.

The differential diagnosis at various stages of the course of this disease includes:

- Colic
- Abdominal strongylosis
- Tetanus
- Azoturia
- Trauma to neck
- Choke
- Grass disease
- Pharyngitis and pharyngeal paralysis
- Lead poisoning

The CPK may rise to 150 000 iu/l or more, while the AST reaches 4500 iu/l plus.

While discussing muscular lesions it is worth remembering the *maxillary myositis* already mentioned as occurring in hyperlipaemia cases, and possibly causing the nutritional check which instigates the hyperlipaemia. Also remember the muscular dystrophy associated with steatitis (yellow fat disease) and sometimes with hyperlipaemia in Shetland and Highland foals and adolescent ponies.

The muscular conditions discussed above need differentiation from muscular-skeletal conditions of the neck and back.

A painful back is usually a localized condition. It is unusual for haematological or biochemical parameters to be affected, except perhaps for moderate rises in CPK and AST if dorsal or lumbar muscles are involved. There is a tendency for the back to be somewhat, if only slightly, arched, and there is always a reluctance to dip the back suddenly or to bend comfortably in a lateral direction. When made to turn in its own length the horse moves awkwardly and all in one piece.

A painful neck used to be relatively common in horses, and there were three main causes:

(1) *Tuberculosis* (bovine) affecting the third, fourth, fifth or sixth intervertebral joints.
(2) *Brucellosis* (*abortus*) affecting the fourth to the sixth intervertebral joints, or the joints between the seventh cervical and first dorsal vertebrae, and the heads of the first ribs.

(3) *Trauma* – usually resulting from a fall on the landing side of a
    jump with a head and neck momentarily forced laterally
    onto the ground by the weight of the falling horse. Here
    again the damage is usually to the intervertebral joints in the
    lower portion of the neck.

Of the three aetiological possibilities trauma is likely to be the
most painful, and diagnosis may be assisted by signs of soft
tissue injury. As time goes on, however, these disappear
leaving osteoarthritic intravertebral changes to produce permanent disability. Tuberculosis is very rare today, and could be
forgotten were it not for the increase in incidence of bovine
tuberculosis in several areas of Britain. Some years ago
brucellosis was relatively common as a cause of this type of
lesion, but the condition is now very rare in cattle, and therefore
very rare also in the horse.

All three possibilities produce much the same clinical picture.
The horse finds it difficult to reach the floor to graze, and may
not be able to drink to the bottom of its bucket. When necessary
it straddles its forelegs either fore and aft, or laterally, in the
effort to graze and drink. When the head and neck are pulled
laterally as if to turn the horse in its own length there is pain,
unless the horse can move its hindquarters in the opposite
direction to keep its long axis straight. Stand the animal against
a wall, and turn its head and neck towards you while pressing
its shoulders against the wall with your free hand. This
produces obvious signs of pain, sometimes more marked when
the head and neck are pulled to one side rather than the other.

Lateral radiography may be very useful particularly in trauma
cases, while the tuberculin test, vague as it is in horses, and the
Brucella abortus serum agglutination test may be helpful too.

15 Lameness

The clinical approach
Special conditions
   Sporadic lymphangitis
   Weanling disease
   'Avonmouth disease' – lead/zinc toxicity

This Chapter is not intended as an exhaustive survey of lameness in the horse and pony, but rather as a guide to the clinical approach in lameness cases. Lameness may be defined simply as an impediment in gait. It may, of course, be painful or non-painful, for it is occasionally purely mechanical. Nevertheless, by common usage, lameness is interpreted as involving some degree of pain. The type of lameness varies according to the work pattern of the horse – many lamenesses are occupational hazards. Steeplechasers, hunters, polo ponies and draught horses all have tendencies to their own classes of lameness. *In general in riding horses and children's ponies the site of lameness, particularly in the forelimb, is more likely to be in the foot than anywhere else.* It is a good rule, in cases where there is nothing obvious to see or feel, to search the foot, and if nothing is found, to search the foot again. And possibly again! And if one is certain that the site of lameness *is* the foot, suspect pus until absolutely certain otherwise. These rules are very old and very sound, and are really the beginning and the end of the diagnosis and treatment of equine lameness.

In lame horses, always suspect the foot until proven otherwise. In foot lameness always suspect pus until proven otherwise. If there is pus let it out: otherwise let him rest.

Remember that a lame horse is a clinical case in no way different from any other clinical case, and the same procedure applies. Above all, take your time. It is quite impossible to assess a lame horse properly in a hurry. Watch it standing quietly at rest: then moving quietly on a halter or head collar. Assess its general demeanour. Is it worried, or in severe pain? Or is the lame leg no more than a minor inconvenience? Obtain a full history just as one would for any other disease. How old is the patient? What work does it do? How long ago did it go lame? When was it last shod? By whom? What type of shoe was used? Did the lameness develop insidiously or suddenly? If suddenly, what was the horse doing when it happened? Is it getting worse? Does rest help, or does the lameness get more severe with inactivity? Has it happened before?

Take careful note of any visible wound, swelling or noticeable difference between the legs. Does it stand square on its front legs. If it shifts weight from one foot to the other, or stands with one fore foot advanced then it may have navicular disease. Don't touch! Look! A severely pus-affected foot may be so painful that the horse cannot keep it still, and keeps lifting it, then touching it to the ground. A horse with a painful shoulder may let the leg hang just behind the vertical with the dorsal wall of the hoof just touching the ground. The pony with laminitis stands with its hindlimbs well under it, and the forelegs in front of the vertical. It may rock slowly back on to its hindquarters with the toe of the front shoes not quite taking weight.

Then have the horse walked away from you for 20 yards or so, turned, and brought back, making certain that it is allowed a good 18 inches of headrope. Make sure also that the groom keeps the horse between him and the examining clinician when turning to come back. Then the horse should be trotted away, turned and trotted back. Not too fast. One learns far more at a collected and balanced trot than when the horse and groom are both extended. While it trots away watch the quarters: if it is slightly lame on a hindleg the quarter on the lame side is carried higher than the sound one. If, however, a horse is *very* lame on a hindleg the quarter of that leg may actually sink as the leg tries to take the weight. Learn to quantify the degree of lameness – it may sound irrelevant but it does help to give the lameness a number, e.g. 2/10 lame on the left fore. When the horse is trotting towards you watch the head – it lowers its head as it takes weight on the sound foreleg. Some clinicians tend to think of the movement as raising the head, or holding the head higher as the painful foreleg takes weight. The ground surface upon which you examine the horse must be hard and smooth, but not slippery. A road or metalled track makes the best surface for such an examination.

Watch particularly carefully as the horse turns as some types of front foot lameness show up very clearly during this movement. Laminitis is such a condition. These manoeuvres concluded, it is advisable to trot the horse across your front, so that you can observe the length of stride and notice any check during the stifle flexion, often a sign of a slight degree of upward fixation of the patella. You can also observe how the feet are placed on the ground, e.g. horses with bone spavin may dig the toe in as the hind foot is placed on the ground, whilst laminitis cases may prefer to take the weight of their front feet back towards the heel. Finally make the horse turn in its own length in both directions. If in doubt about back, or high hindlimb lameness it should be backed for a few paces. Do not make the mistake, when dealing with a horse lame on a hindlimb, of assuming that it is lame on the opposite foreleg!

By now one is aware of the lame leg. Look well at it. Look for inflammatory swellings, cuts and bruises, oedema, and joint enlargement, particularly of knees and fetlocks. Look for sandcracks, false quarters, laminitis rings, and swellings at the coronet indicative of exostoses within the foot itself. If there are no visible lesions in a foreleg it is probable that the site of lameness is in the foot or shoulder. In the hindlimb the foot and the hock are the more usual sites for lameness. Stand in front of each hock in turn, i.e. at a point lateral to the shoulder, and look at its medial silhouette, comparing it with the silhouette on the other side. Look for thickening across the stifle joint, for fluid swelling just anteriomedial to this joint. Only when the lame limb has been methodically examined visually should one approach the horse closely to handle the limb. Any visible abnormality should be checked out first before proceeding to the rest of the leg, but unless such a visible abnormality is very obviously the site of lameness, the rest of the leg should also be checked. It is quite possible, for example, for a horse with a visible, but old and healing tendon lesion to have pus in the foot.

Once any visible abnormality has been checked carefully by palpation, the rest of the lame leg must be examined meticulously. *Start with the foot.* The sole must be thoroughly cleaned with a hoof knife, and all suspicious areas investigated. All cavities, and sites where the horn is obviously degenerate must be trimmed out until healthy horn is reached, or until it is established that infection has reached sensitive tissue. Obviously the first possibility to check is the presence or otherwise of a foreign body, e.g. a flint or nail. (In this connection it is worth reminding your clients at every opportunity that if they pull a nail or spike out of the sole while riding, they must mark the site of entry in some way, e.g. scratching a circle around it with a penknife. Otherwise, when the horse is presented to you some hours, or even some days later, it may not be easy to find the nail hole.) If the horse is shod the shoe should be checked to ensure: (1) that it is not too tight, i.e. binding (the nails too close to sensitive tissue), and (2) that the horse has not been pricked, i.e. the nail has actually touched sensitive tissue. In either case the clenches are likely to be set very high. Alternatively the shoe may be worn and loose, or have twisted on the foot. An ill-fitting shoe with the inner heel set too close often produces a corn, particularly on the front foot. The web of the shoe may well hide infected nail holes, or the toe obscure a seedy toe lesion. It is obvious that the foot cannot be examined properly with the shoe still in place, and yet to remove a shoe and find nothing will cause the owner much time and expense in getting the shoe replaced. Nevertheless if the clinician has good grounds for the belief that the foot is the site of the lameness then he must convince the owner of the wisdom of removing the shoe.

The possibility of laminitis must never be overlooked. The shape of the front wall, the presence of 'seedy toe', the convexity of the sole, and the presence of a pulse in the digital vessels, either above or below the fetlock, all help in confirming a diagnosis. In longstanding cases the ringed and concave front wall is very helpful, as is radiography from the lateral position. In recent acute cases solar haemorrhages may be very useful, occurring as they do over the point of the pedal bone and along the white lines. The wall must be checked for sandcracks, ground cracks, false quarter, etc., and the cornet examined carefully for bony swelling due, for example, to pyramidal disease, sidebone, low ringbone, etc.

If a complete physical and manual examination of the foot has revealed nothing of significance, and particularly if, in a forefoot, there is evidence of contraction, or evidence that the lameness is bilateral, then radiography for navicular disease may be carried out. Radiography may also reveal pedal osteitis. If there is uncertainty as to whether lameness is bilateral or not, it is worth performing a high plantar block on the lame limb, when the opposite limb will appear to be the lame one in bilateral cases.

All parts of the lame leg from the coronet upwards should be handled, searching for new bone, soft tissue swelling, synovial distension and tendon injury. The foot must be lifted and in the foreleg the pastern, fetlock and knee joints fully flexed and fully extended looking for pain and restriction of movement. The elbow should be fully flexed, and as much shoulder movement obtained as is possible. In the hindleg full flexion and extension of the pastern, fetlock and hock is checked, and the spavin test carried out. This involves the horse being held by an attendant at the beginning of a suitable 20 years or so of road or track. The operator then holds the affected hindlimb in full flexion for a complete minute. He must ensure that he grips the lower third of the metatarsal area when flexing the limb – this avoids involving the fetlock and pastern joints. After the full minute the horse is encouraged to trot away smartly, and if active bone spavin is present it will be significantly lame for the first two to three paces. On the whole more information about the hip and stifle are gained during the initial visual examination than during the full examination, but an effort should be made to obtain as much movement in these joints as possible.

Upward fixation of the patella is fairly common in ponies. The patella fails to disengage itself from its position on the extended stifle joint and so flexion cannot occur. The condition may be unilateral or bilateral. There is possibly a hereditary disposition as it occurs more commonly in straight-legged horses. However it also occurs in young horses in poor bodily condition and may be associated with a lack of fat padding out the stifle area. The condition may show an acute form when the patella will not come free and the leg is locked in extension. The leg is straight and the toe drags along the ground. The patella may free itself and the stifle jerk into flexion only for the condition to recur a few paces later. Most cases are much less acute and all that happens is that the patella catches as the pony walks, and frees itself immediately giving a jerky flexion. This may occur at every pace or only intermittently. If the clinician walks beside the pony with his hand on the stifle he can feel the click as the patella frees itself into flexion.

Iliac thrombosis is characterized by complete normality at rest, or at quiet walking or slow trotting paces, but at a steady trot on the lunge a gradual deterioration occurs. First the horse becomes slightly lame on the affected hindleg, but as time goes on the leg becomes quite unusable and the patient, obviously in considerable pain, pulls up three legged, with the affected leg held stiffly away from the body with the foot off the ground. The horse may be sweating profusely apart from this leg, and the pulse in the affected leg is weak, thready or practically non-existent. When allowed to rest there is marked discomfort for some minutes, possibly due to acute 'pins and needles' in the affected limb as the blood supply passes the thrombosed area in sufficient quantity to catch up with the demand.

Conditions causing lameness meriting special consideration

Sporadic lymphangitis (originally known as weed, shakes or Monday morning leg)

The typical disease affected heavy draught horses which were kept on a highly nitrogenous diet, e.g. peans and beans, over a rest period – usually the weekend. It was believed that the disease was due to histamine release, presumably associated with toxic products of digestion in the gut. *Symptoms* included a high temperature with a rapid pulse and rapid respirations, and muscular tremors. Acute lameness developed very quickly in a hindlimb, sometimes in both hindlimbs, or rarely in a forelimb. The affected hindlimb was held in an abducted position with the toe just touching the ground. The inguinal lymphatic nodes were swollen and painful, and most of the limb was swollen, tense and oedematous. The lymphatic vessels stood out like tense cords down the inside of the leg and the skin oozed transudate which led to hair loss. After a few days the oozing glistening limb began to improve, but further attacks tended to occur, and after several attacks the leg was left permanently thickened due to fibrous change. *The typical form of the disease is rarely seen today, but milder and more localized forms appear in ponies and hunters, often when the grass is rich and young. The hock alone, and sometimes the whole leg, is affected.*

Weanling disease (bone dystrophy; idiopathic rickets)

This condition tends to affect Thoroughbreds and half-breds from foalhood up to about 2 years old. Sufferers are usually on good grass and heavily fed. It seems that protein levels are too high, and the young animals grow too fast. Calcium intake tends to be too low, and phosphorus intake too high. There may be excess phosphorus in the urine. Sometimes the disease is related to excess bran in the feed, as was 'Miller's disease' in cart-horse days. In effect, the animal outgrows its mineral intake. The epiphyseal lines as seen on radiography become open, ragged and woolly. There are painful epiphyseal swellings, causing lameness. The pasterns become too upright, while pastern and fetlock joints knuckle forwards. New bone is laid down at the lower end of the radii, and on the sesamoid bones. Many cases, however, are considerably less severe, and are only slightly lame with new bone laid down particularly near the joints.

'Avonmouth' disease – lead/zinc toxicity

This condition is seen in older foals and yearlings in specific areas, usually the fall-out areas of heavy industry, where both zinc and lead levels in the soil and herbage are high. In these circumstances, although the lead level in blood and tissues becomes high enough to cause toxicity in its own right, the interaction between lead and zinc in the body produces an enhanced picture of zinc toxicity without signs of lead poisoning as such. There is retardation of growth, and anaemia, but the important symptoms are orthopaedic in nature, involving swelling at the epiphyses of all the long bones producing widespread pain, stiffness and lameness. The animal becomes tucked up with a somewhat arched back, and very straight legs. Fetlocks and pasterns are enlarged, straight and painful. Hocks and knees are also enlarged, with considerable new bone formation. The youngster spends much time in lateral recumbency and finds difficulty in rising to its feet. There is increased synovial fluid in the affected joints.

16 Skin diseases

Parasites and bacteria
  Lice
  Ringworm
  Chorioptic mange and sarcoptic mange
  Harvest mites
  Dermatophilus infections
  Hyperkeratosis of the ear
  Acne
  Parafilaria
  Oxyuris
  'Warbles'
Allergic conditions
  Urticaria
  Contact allergy
Neoplasia
  Papillomas
  Sarcoids
  Melanomas
  Carcinomas
  Lymphosarcomas
Miscellaneous skin conditions
  Nodular disease
  Vitiligo
  Cutaneous asthenia
  Greasy heel
  Cushing's disease
  Photosensitization
  Biliary obstruction

A surprisingly large number of skin diseases affect the horse. The following is by no means an exhaustive list, but is intended to include those most likely to appear in equine work in Britain.

Parasites and bacteria

Lice

Lice are very common, particularly in the months of January and February. They cause pruritis and hair loss, and are particularly common in hairy poorly groomed ponies kept in relatively crowded conditions. Infested animals bite and rub themselves quite severely. Lice are most easily found just beneath the mane, in the submaxillary space, and above the tail head. Use a fine-toothed comb and a magnifying glass, if necessary, and look carefully for the parasite and its eggs.

Ringworm

Ringworm is also very common in horses in this country, and is highly contagious, particularly to foals and adolescent horses. Both trichophyton and microsporon species infest horses: the microsporon lesion looks like a small papule, very similar in shape and size to the so-called 'humour' papule already mentioned under allergic conditions (p. 95). The superficial covering becomes a tiny scab or scale, and when picked off, a tiny reddish ulcer is seen underneath. The lesion of trichophyton species is larger, up to 1 or 2 inches (2.5–5 cm) in diameter. It appears as a circular area of slightly raised skin with broken hairs sticking through it. When the edge of the circle is lifted it can be peeled off leaving a damp circular pink area underneath – more deeply coloured round the perimeter than in the pale and drier centre. Unfortunately ringworm lesions are not always as easy as this to recognize, as some of the trychophyton species produce irregularly shaped and sized lesions with greyish crusts. When in doubt it is worthwhile producing a lifted lesion or scraping for laboratory culture. If doubt still remains it is better to treat.

Mange

Chorioptic mange

This is much less common than in the days of the heavy horse with hairy heels. It causes 'itchy heel'. The affected animal stamps, kicks and attempts to rub its heel on the other hindleg or against a suitable post. The condition is still seen in half-bred animals and cobs with hairy heels. The lesions are exudative at first, but eventually hard asbestos-like crusts develop which are difficult to deal with. There is no difficulty in finding mites.

Sarcoptic mange

This is now almost extinct in the horse; it produces small hairless patches which exude serum and form scabs. Pruritis is severe. Most lesions occur on the neck and shoulder, but they can occur anywhere. Deep skin scrapings are required for diagnosis as in other species.

Harvest mites

These mites can cause great irritation to thin-skinned horses, e.g. Thoroughbreds, in the late summer and early autumn months, when they cause exudative lesions on the pasterns. This condition is mainly seen on the white areas of the legs – rarely on dark skin.

Dermatophilus congolense infections (mycotic dermatitis)

This organism is believed to be responsible for various lesions of the horse. These include rain scald, mud fever and cracked heels. Rain scald develops along the back following a long period of wet weather. The hair and skin of grazing horses – particularly those with long and matted hair – becomes saturated and dirty, ideal for the development of this organism. Pieces, roughly oval, of skin lift and can be peeled off leaving a wet patch smeared with pus. The peeled-off top has a tuft of hair sticking up from it. In the heel, and behind the pastern up to the fetlock exudate forms, mats the hair, and forms scabs. Deep cracks often form in the heel in a transverse direction with much swelling and considerable pain. Secondary bacterial invasion prolongs healing. In very wet muddy conditions sores with exudate may form up the inside of the hindleg into the inguinal region and even forward along the ventral abdomen. The organism can be cultured on blood agar from fresh lesions, but in older lesions it is better to make smears and stain with methylene blue to show up the typical mycelium.

Hyperkeratosis of the ear pinna

Occasionally a horse will show whitish or yellowish-white plaques, slightly raised from the level of the surrounding pinna. Most such lesions do not affect the horse, but some cause irritation and head shaking. The condition may be due to the fly simulium.

Acne/botriomycosis

Staphylococcal skin infections occasionally occur in horses as in other animals. The organism infects the hair follicles and may cause abscesses ('boils'). Quite a number of these boils may form at the same time in dirty horses, or in stables where the saddlery and other fomites are dirty.

Chronic staphylococcal granulomas may also occur in horses. One site is the spermatic cord at castration: the other is at the front of the shoulder in draught horses where the collar is continually rubbing against the skin.

Parafilaria multipapillosa

This is an Eastern European and Russian disease in which adult filarial worms living just beneath the skin stimulate small soft skin swellings over the shoulders and chest. In temperatures above 60°F (15.5°C) the worm penetrates the skin and discharges eggs and microfilaria in a small trickle of blood. Blood-sucking vectors, of types not present in Britain, pass infection on to new hosts. Transmission does not occur in this country and the disease is seen only in recently imported horses.

Oxyuris equi

This parasite causes intense perianal irritation due to the females at the anus laying their eggs on the perineum. The horse rubs its tail against any solid object, and causes bare patches at the tail base and in some cases injury to the skin. Female worms and eggs can be seen on the anus: the appearance of large number of eggs adherent to the perineum is known as 'rust'.

Warbles

Warbles are practically unknown in horses today following the eradication programme in cattle. When they do occur, the parasite under the skin of the horse's back is not capable of a full life history: the 'warble' on the back is usually small and deformed, and the parasite within incapable of continuing the life cycle. Do not attempt to squeeze it out of the warble swelling for if the larva is crushed beneath the skin an anaphylactic reaction may occur. It is better to leave it alone, or at the most apply hot fomentations.

Allergic conditions

(1) Urticaria (see p. 95).
(2) Contact allergies (see p. 95).

Neoplasia

Papillomas

Papillomas (warts) are seen frequently in young horses from 6 months to 24 months of age. They are usually profusely spread over the muzzle and lips. Of small size, they look like the warts seen on the back of children's hands. They are of virus origin and disappear spontaneously in a few months.

Sarcoids

Sarcoids are the most common tumours found in adult horses. They are fibroblastic tumours with a tendency to malignancy, and they are probably of primary viral aetiology. They originate as hard nodules of fibrous material which erode through the superficial skin layers, and then tend to look like granulation tissue. Surgical removal tends to stimulate the development of further sarcoids in the immediate area.

Melanomas

These neoplasms with a high tendency to malignancy are seen particularly on grey horses, and become more common in middle and old age. They are specially found on the perineum around the anus, on the hairless ventral areas of the tail, and on the vulva, and prepuce. They sometimes occur within the anus on the rectal wall. They are also seen, occasionally, on the head and neck, the folds of the flank, and rarely elsewhere on the body. Care must be taken to avoid these lesions being abraded or crushed, for malignant 'flare-ups' may occur.

Carcinomas

Squamous cell carcinomas occur at several external sites. The most common is the third eyelid, where the lesion looks like slowly growing granulation tissue. If not removed it spreads to the eyelids and skin of the face. Similar lesions occur occasionally on the vulva and scrotum. They are malignant, but fortunately do not metastasize quickly.

Cutaneous lymphosarcomas (see p. 37)

These lesions may initially be confused with the lesions of nodular disease.

Miscellaneous skin lesions

Nodular disease – necrobiosis

This disease is seen relatively frequently. The nodules are up to a centimetre, sometimes a little more, in size, and occur in the dermis over the back, the sides of the chest, and the shoulder. They cause the horse no harm, except that it is unwise to fit saddlery or harness over affected areas as they may become abraded. The condition is probably an allergic one producing collagen degeneration; some lesions necrose involving the overlying epidermis, producing hairless areas of skin which may show scarring. The condition is then called 'nodular necrobiosis'. This complication is much less likely to occur if saddlery and clothing are avoided.

Vitiligo

This is simply a loss of pigment from hair and skin in limited areas of the body, generally about the head. The condition is harmless apart from its unsightliness, and in most cases is probably traumatic in origin.

Cutaneous asthenia (the Ehlers–Danlos syndrome)

This is a hereditary, congenital, primary connective tissue dysplasia most severe in man, dogs, cats, cattle and sheep. It is much milder in pigs and horses. The disease affects the collagen content of the skin, but in the horse the diseased skin areas are localized rather than total, and while the affected skin is fragile and tears more easily than normal the extent of the lesions produced is limited.

Greasy heel (seborrhoea)

This disease was largely seen in cart-horses with hairy heels, and is only seen today in horses carrying a great deal of feather. It was usually seen in heels already affected by chorioptes. There was exudation of greasy seborrhoeic material in the heel which matted the hair and predisposed to bacterial infection.

Cushing's disease (hyperadrenocorticism)

Cushing's disease is uncommon, but does occasionally occur. There is polyuria, polydypsia, loss of weight, with a pendulous abdomen. Hair loss may occur in some areas; other cases will show areas of more profuse hair growth. Temperature, pulse rate and respirations remain normal.

Photosensitization

See Chapter 6.

Biliary obstruction

In cases involving severe biliary obstruction, as in some cases of pancreatic neoplasia, pruritic wet eczematous lesions with hair loss may occur on the coronets and lower legs (see Chapter 6).

17 The udder

Mastitis

The equine udder is relatively trouble free, and it is unusual to meet serious mastitis. Usually mastitis is streptococcal in origin, particularly *Strep. zooepidemicus*, and responds rapidly to penicillin group antibiotics. The udder is hot, swollen, tense and painful, and there is quite marked and extensive oedema. The mare is often lethargic and her hindquarter movement is stiff. The milk is usually thickened, and may be discoloured and contain clots. The oedema may make it quite difficult to withdraw milk for bacteriology, or to strip the udder prior to antibiotic treatment. It may be necessary to bathe the udder with warm water before stripping, which should be performed several times daily. It is usually possible to introduce the nozzle of the intramammary antibiotic tube into the largest of the teat ducts – force must not be used. If not, parenteral treatment will be necessary, and may be helpful in any event.

It is worth remembering that the udder immediately after weaning may be hot, swollen and painful, and will benefit from bathing and long-acting antibiotic therapy.

Confusion also occurs in the days immediately post-foaling, when, again, the udder may be swollen and oedematous to the extent that the mare may resent the foal's attempts to drink. Once again, bathing and hand stripping may help until the swelling and oedema are somewhat reduced.

18 Peracute diseases, sudden death and 'found dead' syndromes

Sudden death and 'found dead'
    Haemorrhage
    Acute cardiac failure
    Electrocution
    Lightning strike
    Yew poisoning
    Water dropwort
Peracute diseases
    Acute anaphylactic shock
    Purpura
    Anthrax
    Acute enteritis
    Torsion of the small gut
    Leptospirosis
    Botulism
    Peracute grass disease
    Polymyositis
    Wound gas gangrene (malignant oedema)
    Hypocalcaemia
    Transit tetany

Sudden death and 'found dead' syndromes

Comparatively few diseases actually cause sudden death in the horse. Yet as far as the horse owner is concerned if he leaves his horse alone and apparently healthy, and on his return next day the horse is dead, he always reports it as a case of sudden death, although the course of the illness might have been nearly 24 hours, or even longer if the horse was already showing slight and unnoticed symptoms when seen the day before. Hence the distinction, for in fact many apparently sudden death cases are cases of peracute or even acute disease. True causes of sudden death include:

Haemorrhage

This may be *external*, e.g. from a stake wound in the lower neck or the chest, or *internal*, e.g. from a *ruptured splenic haematoma*, or from an *aortic rupture*. These haemorrhages usually occur during exercise. The aorta usually ruptures close to the aortic valves.

Acute cardiac failure

Electrocution

Lightning strike

Yew poisoning

This may be so sudden that the horse still has yew leaves in its mouth. It is usually possible to find pieces of yew in its stomach. There may be brief convulsions before death. Any surviving horses will show colicky pain and diarrhoea. All parts of the yew tree are poisonous, whether fresh or old.

Water dropwort

Rare in horses, but the tubers are as toxic in the horse as in cattle, and are usually eaten when they are dug up during ditching operations and left on the grass close to the ditch. Symptoms include abdominal pain, salivation, muscular spasms and convulsions, leading to death within a few minutes of onset. Sublethal doses cause a greenish diarrhoea.

Peracute disease

Anaphylactic shock

Subnormal temperature, wildly beating heart, very fast pulse, cold clammy body surfaces, some sweating, dyspnoea with rapid respiratory movements. Most cases recover, developing extensive oedematous plaques over the body surface during the recovery phase. The plaques disappear in 24–36 hours.

Purpura haemorrhagica

An acute anaphylactic reaction believed to be associated with streptococcal infection. Massive oedema of skin, lungs and gut. Extensive haemorrhages. (See Chapter 13.)

Anthrax

May need differentiation from purpura. There is usually an initial high temperature up to 106°F (41°C) which drops as the disease progresses. Respirations and pulse rate are very rapid. The horse looks very ill, will not eat, is colicky, and tense hot swellings caused by inflammatory exudate and oedema appear on its neck, throat and chest, interfering with respiration. There may be similar swellings of the sheath and mammary glands. These swellings are not invariably present. There is an acute enteritis, there is often diarrhoea, which may be blood stained. Death may occur from septicaemia, but often results from asphyxia and toxaemia before septicaemia supervenes. Blood smears are not, therefore, always satisfactory for confirmation of diagnosis. A smear may be taken of exudate from an incision into a typical external swelling, or a small incision into the abdomen may be made, with care, to obtain a swab of peritoneal fluid for examination for anthrax organisms.

Acute enteritis

Clostridium difficile or *Cl. perfringens* B – salmonellosis (see Chapter 4).

Torsion of the small intestine

This condition (amongst other abdominal catastrophies) may easily kill within a few hours (see Chapter 2).

Leptospirosis

See Chapter 6.

Botulism

See Chapter 10.

Peracute grass disease

Temperature in normal range, pulse rate 80 plus, profuse sweating behind shoulders and in front of stifles, pendulous penis, dysphagia, muscular tremors, regurgitation of green fluid from stomach down nose with painful antiperistaltic movements of oesophagus. Rapid dehydration and haemoconcentration occurs. Complete gut atony with colonic impaction and abdominal pain. No faeces passed.

Polymyositis

See Chapter 14.

Wound gas gangrene (malignant oedema)

Caused by the invasion of anaerobic and tissue-damaged wounds by the organism *Clostridium septique*. Castration wounds are very prone to this infection in horses. Toxaemia and death can occur within 24 hours of operation. The lesion may look almost insignificant, merely a few strands of reddened, gelatinous, and crepitating material in the scrotum or the cord.

Hypocalcaemia

See Chapter 20.

Transit tetany

See Chapter 20.

19 Pyrexia of unknown origin

Septicaemia
Anthrax
Pneumonia
Laminitis
Endocarditis
Abscess
Brucellosis
Viraemia

This confusing syndrome is not unusual in horses. Strictly speaking the phrase implies that there are no clinical signs apart from a significantly raised temperature with resultant lethargy, lowered appetite, and other signs relating to the temperature. The clinical problem is to appreciate the appearance of signs which will indicate the cause of the high temperature, and sooner or later these always appear. In fact they are often present at the outset if one looks hard enough. The origin of the pyrexia may only be unknown because the clinician did not find it; nevertheless these cases are often very confusing.

Septicaemia

There is usually a period at the onset of a septicaemic condition when pyrexia is the only indication. Within 24 hours some degree of localization may occur and signs of diarrhoea, or pneumonia, for example, may appear. The diarrhoea of salmonellosis may well follow 12–18 hours of high temperature, congested mucous membranes, rising pulse rate, ending with a varying degree of abdominal pain with colicky symptoms. There is usually leucopenia and neutropenia. When diarrhoea supervenes the pulse may rise even further, but the temperature drops. Leucopenia and neutropenia may give way to leucocytosis and neutrophilia. Streptococcal septicaemias may last considerably longer than salmonella septicaemias before any localization occurs.

Anthrax

This is often not septicaemic in the horse, but there is usually a high temperature at the beginning of its course. In 8–12 hours, however, the abdominal pain, scanty blood-stained diarrhoea, and hot painful inflammatory swellings around the throat, neck and chest, have at least begun to appear.

Pneumonia

Pneumonia in the horse may cause a temperature of 104–105°F (40–40.5°C) for some 12 hours before typical signs appear. In the preliminary congestive phase there may be a rapid respiratory rate, a raised pulse and congested mucous membranes. When pneumonic signs and sounds appear the temperature usually becomes lower.

Laminitis

Some cases of acute laminitis show a preliminary high temperature, as high as 105°F (40.5°C) at the onset of clinical signs. There will be rapid respirations, anxiety and a high pulse rate, and at this stage a misdiagnosis of acute respiratory disease may be made. Within a matter of hours, however, a strong digital pulse, hot coronets, painful feet, and the typical laminitic stance will have begun to develop.

Endocarditis

This relatively rare condition of the horse may be very confusing. Initially there is often a lengthy period of pyrexia, which may vary in degree, but does not disappear. It may last for as long as 3 months and during this period there is shifting lameness, and some loss of weight. Shifting lameness should always make one suspicious of endocarditis. Gradually developing anaemia and a degree of lethargy may also occur. Respirations may be slightly accelerated, but do not attract immediate attention. Antibiotic treatment causes temporary lowering of temperature, but does not significantly affect the pulse rate, which stays at 50–60 per minute. Eventually oedema of the legs occurs. At some stage during this clinical progression a cardiac murmur will be noticed. Haematology reveals anaemia, leucocytosis and neutrophilia.

Abscess

An encapsulated abscess, particularly one sited in an internal lymphatic node, may produce a long period of pyrexia, temporarily responsive to antibiotics, but always recurring. Such an abscess may eventually rupture to set up pyaemia, but it seems possible that in some cases after extensive antibiotic treatment massive encapsulation occurs, and the clinical picture resolves.

Brucellosis

Brucellosis is rare now that it has to all intents and purposes been eradicated in the cattle population. The disease takes several clinical forms in the horse. It may affect the synovial bursae – particularly the occipital or the supraspinous bursae producing poll-evil or fistulous withers. It may affect the intravertebral cervical joints in the lower part of the neck producing a stiff neck (see Chapter 14). It occasionally affects a limb joint, or tendon sheaths in the legs.

But the syndrome under consideration at the moment is the 'undulant fever' syndrome, producing an intermittent temperature with muscle pain and stiffness and great depression. Anaemia may develop. Aspartate aminotransferase (AST), creatine phosphokinase (CPK), total serum proteins and globulin usually rise. Diagnosis is by the serum agglutination test, the complement fixation test, and Coombs test. A serum antibody test (SAT) reading of above 2/40 (60 iu/ml); a complement function test (CFT) reading of above 1/40, or a Coombs test (AGT) reading of 4/160 are regarded as positive.

Viraemia

It seems possible that several viruses, probably of respiratory groupings, are able to produce ongoing viraemia syndromes in the horse without further symptoms developing. There is, however, very little firm evidence that this is the case. The possibility should not be neglected when dealing with cases of pyrexia of unknown origin in the horse. Blood pictures showing anaemia, leucopenia, neutropenia, lymphocytosis and monocytosis may be suggestive.

20 Diseases producing nervous symptoms

Hypocalcaemia
Transit tetany
Synchronous diaphragmatic flutter
Hepatic encephalopathy
Uraemia
Lead poisoning
Bracken poisoning
Heat stroke
Tetanus
Botulism
Polymyositis
Louping-ill
Rabies
Listeriosis
Space-occupying lesions in the brain
The 'falling' horse
Localized nervous symptoms
    Facial nerve paralysis
    Trigeminal nerve paralysis
    Equine herpes virus paresis
    The wobbler syndrome
    Neuritis of the cauda equina
    Head flicking

This group is not confined to primary diseases of the nervous system itself. From the clinician's viewpoint it must include conditions in which the clinical picture suggests neurological disease even if the aetiology is not primarily neurological.

Hypocalcaemia

Hypocalcaemia in the mare is eclamptic in nature, and is not necessarily immediately postparturient. It often occurs weeks or even a month or so after parturition, at a time when the foal's appetite for milk is very high. The syndrome shows initial apprehension and restlessness followed by sweating. Then comes a fixed staring expression, with rapid respirations, and an unsteady stiff-legged gait. There is a degree of trismus. Pulse rate is high and the mare is unable to swallow, very anxious and excitable. Faeces are scanty or absent. Finally collapse and convulsive movements occur ending in coma. At various stages during the short course of this disease the symptoms suggest an abdominal catastrophe, an acute respiratory crisis, acute laminitis and tetanus.

Transit tetany

Both calcium and magnesium are involved in this condition which can affect mares during transport by road or rail, particularly if they are lactating or in oestrus. It also affects ponies of either sex, including geldings. Undue and prolonged fatigue even without a journey may also precipitate the condition. The first signs are tetanic spasms of most superficial muscles, particularly the masseters; muscular tremors, marked trismus and a stiff-legged gait. Temperature remains normal unless the animal is very excited, but pulse and respirations are very rapid. There is profuse sweating, anxiety and distress, followed by collapse and convulsive struggling. The early stages of this disease look very much like early tetanus, but in transit tetany the membrana nictitans is not involved.

Synchronous diaphragmatic flutter

A puzzling condition for the clinician, tending to occur in exhausted horses which are, or have been, sweating profusely, although it may happen in horses sweating profusely for other reasons. The condition is believed to be associated with low blood levels of calcium and potassium. The syndrome involves contractions of the diaphragm synchronous with the heart beat. To the onlooker the horse seems to be undergoing a series of exhausting 'hiccups'. It is always worth treating such cases with slow intravenous calcium borogluconate, for the manner in which the condition disappears during treatment is diagnostic.

Hepatic encephalopathy (see p. 55)

This may easily be confused with a primary cerebral condition such as cerebral neoplasia, or increased intracranial pressure due, for example, to 'dropsy of the lateral ventricles'.

Uraemia

Seen in particular in terminal renal failure due to advanced kidney disease (see p. 62).

Lead poisoning (see p. 83)

This causes profuse salivation, laryngeal paralysis with snoring, blindness, and aimless wandering with an ataxic gait.

Bracken poisoning

In horses bracken poisoning produces a 'sleepy staggers' syndrome. Bracken is a cumulative poison, and several weeks on bracken-infested pasture are required before symptoms appear. The horse is depressed, stands sleepily with head down and legs spread out. Ataxia develops, then muscular tremors, recumbency, convulsions and death. The course of the disease may last a number of days. The condition in the horse is due to the effect of thiaminase in the bracken, which sets up a thiamine deficiency, and large doses of thiamine, e.g. 1 g daily intravenously or intramuscularly, may be diagnostically useful if given early in the progress of the disease.

Heat stroke

Heat stroke occurs in very high environmental temperatures, particularly in enclosed buildings with high humidity and poor ventilation, especially if there is a shortage of water. Anxiety, tremors, rapid pulse, very high temperature, e.g. 110°F (43°C), and very fast and exaggerated respirations, lead to staggering, frothing at the mouth, collapse and convulsions. Diagnosis depends upon assessment of the temperature rise, and recognition of the environmental factors.

Tetanus

This can be deceptive in the early stages, but it is important to remember that a horse with tetanus nearly always shows tonic spasm of the third eyelid very early in the disease, and that any stimulus causes immediate exacerbation of this sign. It is very easy to produce exaggeration of the tonic spasm by tapping the horse on the nasal peak or forehead with a finger. A little later spasm of the nostrils and lips, and of the skin over the face and head occurs. Trismus is severe, strands of saliva hang from the mouth, and respirations become rapid and shallow due to spasm of the diaphragmatic muscles. The ears become erect and stiff, and the ear tips may, in fact, touch each other over the poll. The eyes are narrowed, the eyelids fixed, and the pupils dilated. These symptoms, along with the dilated nostrils, give an expression of great anxiety characteristic of the disease. A stiff-legged gait follows the earlier signs very rapidly, and leads to complete tonic immobility in a relatively short period of time. The horse stands rigidly with legs spread in the trestle attitude. All the muscles, set in tonic spasm, stand out clearly. The abdomen is tucked up due to contraction of the abdominal muscles; the tail is half erect and quivering, and the penis is partly erect. The pulse rate may be slightly raised. Temperature is usually in normal range, and a rise in temperature is a bad prognostic sign.

Botulism

See Chapter 10.

Polymyositis

See Chapters 10 and 14

Louping-ill

This occurs occasionally in horses and has been recorded in Ireland. The symptoms are variable but include muscular tremors and long periods of recumbency leading to excitement, ataxia and opisthotonus. Diagnosis on clinical grounds alone is obviously very difficult. It might help if there were considerable numbers of sheep in the area, if sheep ticks were prevalent, and if louping-ill occurred among the sheep population, but it is likely that definitive diagnosis could only be made by isolation of the louping-ill virus from the brain and spinal cord at post-mortem examination. Serum antibody levels in life might be helpful, but in a louping-ill area a significant proportion of ponies might be antibody positive, without at any time becoming clinical cases. Histological examination of brain tissue, in the right hands, provides retrospective confirmation.

Rabies

Hopefully rabies will never occur in Great Britain, but it is essential, and may well become increasingly so, that it should be recognized as early as possible should it occur. The affected horse may show unusual behaviour patterns alternating unusual apprehension with marked aggression. It may attempt to bite in an excitable and disorganized manner at a stick held, or moved, in front of its face. Salivation may be evident. There may be extensive muscle tremors followed eventually by posterior paresis, and inability to swallow. Recumbency follows. Occasionally nervous signs may be localized, e.g. as radial paralysis. Any suspicion of rabies should be notified to the Ministry of Agriculture Veterinary Division who will deal with all aspects of the case.

Listeriosis

Listeriosis is still rare in horses, but occurs occasionally in silage-fed animals. Clinical symptoms include pyrexia, weakness and ataxia, with a tendency to circle. Central interference with the seventh and fifth cranial nerves may occur causing facial paralysis, and drooping of the ear and eyelids on the affected side on the one hand, and inability to close the mouth completely on the other (see Chapter 10). Eventually collapse, recumbency and death occur.

Space-occupying lesions in the brain

Such lesions are rare in horses, but when they do occur the clinical picture is similar whatever the lesion. They include cysts, abscesses and aberrant strongyle larvae as well as tumours, e.g. endothelioma. The symptoms are generally mild at onset, slowly getting more severe until collapse, convulsions and coma occur. They include ataxia, head pressing, abnormal stance and aimless wandering. Periods of dullness may alternate with periods of excitability, and may be very difficult to differentiate clinically from lead poisoning, hepatic encephalopathies, advanced uraemic signs, bracken poisoning and other diseases producing central nervous signs. Full use must be made of biochemical investigation for liver and kidney damage, and tests for lead on blood and faeces so as to eliminate as many of the differentials as possible. Hepatic encephalopathies have a high blood ammonia level, but successful estimation of blood ammonia depends on the proximity of a suitable laboratory.

The falling horse

The veterinary surgeon is consulted not infrequently to advise on 'falling' horses, i.e. horses which exhibit transient episodes of collapse, obviously a serious matter for both horse and rider. This syndrome presents one of the most difficult diagnostic problems facing the clinician. It is highly unlikely that he or she will actually witness such an episode – information is nearly always hearsay, often inaccurate, for the episode occurs and is over so quickly that there is often doubt as to what really happened. It is, in fact, seldom that a diagnosis is made. There are several possibilities.

Narcolepsy

This apparently occurs, albeit very occasionally. The horse may suddenly collapse, particularly if excited for any reason, and lie as if paralysed for a period from several seconds to several minutes. The appearance is of flaccid paralysis, but there may be movements of the eyes, tongue or superficial muscles. This type of episode is spoken of as a cataplectic attack, and may occur at varying intervals.

Missed ventricular beats

It is common for horses to exhibit missed ventricular beats from time to time, and this has no particular significance as long as the ventricular beats pick up on exercise. Occasionally the resting horse will miss two or more successive ventricular beats. However, should six or seven successive beats fail to materialize the horse may fall, in which case the impact initiates the full rhythm again and the horse rises dazedly to its feet within a minute or so.

Epileptiform fits

The horse occasionally shows a syndrome clinically similar to the epileptic seizure in the dog – it appears dazed for a second or two and then falls – lying on its side with paddling of all limbs, rapid respirations, some sweating, champing mouth movements with salivation. After a varying period of one or more minutes the horse becomes quiet, and slowly and dazedly gets to its feet.

Localized nervous syndromes

Facial nerve paralysis

See Chapter 12.

Trigeminal nerve paralysis

See Chapter 12.

EHV1 (equine herpes virus) paresis

Horses which have been infected by EHV1 subtype 1 may develop this condition if they are reinfected when their immunity is disappearing. Vascular damage occurs leading to CNS lesions of ischaemic nature. The virus causes pyrexia and varying degrees of respiratory involvement followed by hindquarter incoordination which may lead to paralysis and recumbency.

The wobbler syndrome

Appears in any breed, but mostly in young Thoroughbreds and half-breds from 6 months to 2 years of age, and occasionally in older animals if they have been broken and schooled later in life. The symptoms basically are those of ataxia, affecting the hindlegs largely, and to a much lesser extent in most cases the forelegs. The animal has a swaying gait with placement problems affecting its feet. The hind feet are placed in varying positions on the ground, and in an uncoordinate fashion, whilst the forelegs swing outwards and forwards especially at the trot. The horse may fall if any sudden changes in direction are called for. The condition arises from a point of constriction of the young horse's cord due to a narrowed spinal canal. The usual site is at the level of the third or fourth cervical vertebrae, and may be confirmed by lateral radiography.

Neuritis of the cauda equina

This is a peculiar type of chronic polyneuritis affecting the cauda equina. The lesions develop slowly and are granulomatous in nature. There are a number of hypotheses regarding the aetiology of the condition, but in effect the cause is as yet unknown. The symptoms develop insidiously and include loss of sensation in the perianal area, and the skin of the tail, extending in many cases towards the buttocks and gluteal region. The tail is flaccid and hangs limply, usually wet with urine in the mare. The anus is relaxed, and faeces pass by overflow. The bladder is distended and urine trickles from the vulva or the flaccid penis, wetting the tail in the mare and the hindlegs in the male. The hindleg action may be slightly incoordinate.

Head flicking

There are many possible reasons for head shaking in the horse, but the condition under discussion is not head shaking in the usual sense of the word, but a specific head-flicking syndrome readily recognized. The movement is entirely vertical, and involves a series of quick flicks or jerks which suggest to the observer that the horse has been stung on the end of the nose. It gives the impression in some cases that it is trying to look at its nose-end. The condition may show periods when the flicking becomes much more extravagant, and occasionally the horse rubs its upper lip and nose vigorously against its forelegs, or even walks or trots a few paces with its nose rubbing on the ground. Inspection of the nose, muzzle and mouth is unrewarding, but the condition is almost certainly due to a localized allergic condition. It may occur in stables or at grass, but it is generally more severe in summer than in winter, and it is at its worst on hot, humid summer days, particularly if the horse is pastured where there are groups of trees or tall bushes. Not infrequently the condition improves if the horse is moved to a high open area clear of bushes and trees.

21 The eye

Injuries to the periorbital region and eyelids
Foreign bodies in the eye
Excessive lachrymation
Neoplasms – periorbital region and eyelids
Protrusion of third eyelid
Entropion
Corneal problems
   Scarring
   Keratitis
   Fungal infection
Opacity of lens – cataract
Uveitis
   Iridocyclitis
   Periodic ophthalmia
Retinal haemorrhage

The eye is, in many respects, a subject for the specialist, so there is often reason to consider whether the patient would not be better served by referral to an equine hospital, or to a colleague holding the Diploma in Ophthalmology. Fortunately the majority of cases involving the eye are suffering from lesions of the eyelids, conjunctival membranes or the external surface of the cornea. Lesions of the lens, retina or the aqueous and vitreous humour are relatively uncommon, whilst the most common condition affecting the uveal tract is periodic ophthalmia (recurrent iridocyclitis).

Injuries to the periorbital region and the eyelids are common, varying from minor sclerotic haemorrhage and bruising, with or without laceration of the eyelid, usually the upper, to very extensive damage to the skin and subcutaneous tissues over the supraorbital ridge and the facial region under the eye. Diagnosis is usually uncomplicated, although some cases involving massive anaphylactic response may produce oedematous swelling of the periorbital area, eyelids and conjunctival membranes of similar scale. The absence of contusions, the probability that anaphylactic reactions will be bilateral, and the presence of oedematous plaques in other sites in anaphylactic cases, will aid diagnosis. In fact, most eye lesions of systemic origin are bilateral.

Foreign bodies in the eye are also relatively common in the horse, and may vary in size from small pieces of grit to pieces of twig. The reaction produced varies, but may on occasions produce conjunctival swelling so intense that the cornea is completely hidden. More commonly, it produces blepharospasm, irritation of the cornea, excessive lachrymation, and restlessness. It is not unusual for such foreign bodies to lodge beneath the membrana nictitans, often causing partial protrusion of that organ. Foreign bodies may cause actual damage to the cornea, producing scratches leading to superficial ulceration or even penetration. In neglected cases such lesions may develop to produce panophthalmitis, with swelling of the eyeball, opacity and vascularization of the cornea (pannus), and eventually degeneration and atrophy (phthisis) of the eyeball itself. Rupture is unusual.

There is no merit in attempting more than the most superficial examination of injured or otherwise painful eyes without adequate desensitization by means of local anaesthetic liquid instilled into the affected conjunctival sac. Care should be taken that the third eyelid is adequately desensitized, so that it may be lifted to search underneath. Small foreign bodies, e.g. grit, in contact with the corneal surface may lead to ulceration and a much slower recovery rate. Instillation of fluorescein into the conjunctival sac will allow such foreign bodies and ulcerated areas to be identified much more easily.

Excessive lachrymation from one eye without evidence of irritation or inflammatory reaction may be due to blockage of the nasolachrymal duct. This is easily checked by installing fluorescin into the eye, for in the normal eye the fluorescin will almost immediately appear at the lower end of the duct in the nostril. If this does not happen, the duct may be flushed out by passing a small animal catheter or canula from the nostril end as far up the duct as it will comfortably go before irrigating with a syringe full of saline. A little local anaesthetic ointment will help to facilitate the passage of the catheter by desensitizing the lower opening of the duct.

The periorbital region and the eyelids are prone to neoplastic involvement. It is not unusual for sarcoids to occur along either upper or lower eyelid, although only rarely both, and such lesions, particularly if they involve a canthus, may be very difficult to remove without causing damage and distortion to the lids. Dermoids of congenital origin occasionally occur on the edges of the eyelids, and are also seen on conjunctival and corneal surfaces. Conjunctival sarcomas may occasionally be seen, but the traditional ocular neoplasm of the horse is the squamous cell carcinoma of the third eyelid, occasionally also affecting the main eyelids. Fortunately the lesion does not appear to be highly malignant, and provided that early action is taken, removal of the third eyelid may well be effective. In more advanced cases the whole eye and the conjunctival sac may need removal in the traditional manner. Neglected cases may show metastases in the subparotid lymph node with obvious swelling at that point.

Protrusion of the third eyelid may be seen in tetanus, where it is bilateral, very prominent and one of the earliest signs of the disease. In tetanus protrusion may be momentarily grossly exaggerated by tapping the forehead or the facial bones with the finger end.

A somewhat slack protrusion of the third eyelid may occur in Horner's syndrome, in which the eye sinks into the socket, with pupillary constriction due to sympathetic nerve damage, and drooping of the upper eyelid. Horner's syndrome in the horse is sometimes associated with guttural pouch disease.

Entropion with accompanying trichiasis (i.e. the eyelashes impinging on the cornea) is not infrequently seen in the foal in the first few days of life. In many cases it is transient and temporary, for it usually responds quite well to the suturing together for a few days of two folds of facial skin beneath the lower eyelid. Some equine specialists, however, prefer the surgical removal of a crescentic piece of skin with suturing of the exposed edges as in the dog, while others favour the injection of a bleb of liquid paraffin or intramammary antibiotic ointment into the skin of the lower eyelid as in the lamb.

For accurate and efficient examination of the cornea and deeper structures adequate illumination is necessary. The eye should always be examined in a darkened box; it is impossible to make a satisfactory assessment in daylight. A direct ophthalmo-scope with a wide beam should be used, and the value of one, or preferably two powerful torches should not be underestimated. This is not the place to discuss the technique of using an ophthalmoscope, but it is worth stressing that every opportun-ity should be taken, on whatever pretext, to examine the eyes of normal horses, which show a picture considerably different from that in the dog. In particular the retinal pattern of blood vessels looks almost blurred in comparison. Practice is essential. It is better not to use atropine as a mydriatic, for this drug may cause pupillary dilatation to persist for several days.

It is important to establish that pupillary reaction to light is normal: note that when a bright light is shone into one eye pupillary constriction should occur in both eyes. Difference in pupil size and rate of constriction may indicate a previous attack of periodic ophthalmia with adhesions affecting the iris. Such a difference may also occur in cases of Horner's syndrome.

Examination of the cornea should include a search for corneal scarring resulting from previous trauma, and an assessment of the effect, if any, of such scarring upon the field of vision. The presence or otherwise of ulceration should also be determined. Keratitis may be due to direct trauma, foreign bodies, and/or bacterial infection. Fungal infection also occurs, often as a result of longstanding antibiotic or corticosteroid therapy, and is a very serious complication difficult to treat. In many cases of severe keratitis vascularization of the cornea with pannus formation occurs, gradually fading as healing occurs.

Occasionally, following severe uveitis (iridocyclitis) as occurs in periodic ophthalmia, debris appears in the anterior chamber; fortunately this usually disappears at a varying time after recovery. Pus may collect in the same site after pyogenic infections like strangles.

Opacity of the lens (cataract) is not uncommon in horses,

particularly in middle and old age. It varies very considerably in intensity and distribution, and therefore in its effect on vision. Bilateral cases are obviously graver than unilateral ones, and certainly total severe cataract interferes with sight very considerably. However, there are several causes of cataract including trauma, periodic ophthalmia and old age, and a significant proportion of cases show local and non-progressive lesions that are not very dense. Assessment of the effect upon vision must always be made on an individual basis.

The uveal tract, comprising the iris, the ciliary bodies and the choroid layer, is very important and merits close examination. The tract is a relatively common focus of disease in the horse, and such disease may spread easily to the lens, the retina and even the cornea. It is worth noting that the corpora nigra (black bodies) are extensions from the iris which can be seen protruding into the upper part of the pupillary aperture. They are absolutely normal, with no adverse significance. The veterinary surgeon is frequently consulted by clients who have just noticed the corpora nigra in their own horses, and find their appearance ominous and frightening.

Although various degrees of uveitis are not uncommon in the horse, the most serious disease affecting the uveal tract is that known as periodic ophthalmia, recurrent uveitis, recurrent iridocyclitis or moon blindness. This is an intermittent uveitis which tends to recur. It may affect both eyes, but is often unilateral recurring in the same eye. In the initial acute phase there is pyrexia, profuse lachrymation, depression, and spasm of the eyelids which remain partly closed. There is severe pain and dislike of light. The sclera and conjunctiva are congested, and there may be corneal oedema. The iris is inflamed, and may develop adhesions to the cornea (anterior synechiae) or to the lens (posterior synechiae). The retina may be involved. Symptoms may decrease in severity in a quiescent period preceding a further attack, but corneal opacity, synechiae, and retinal scarring and detachment gradually get worse. Further acute attacks make the position worse until corneal opacity, cataract or optic neuritis eventually lead to blindness. Periodic ophthalmia is believed to be a hypersensitivity disease, possibly associated with leptospiral organisms, although microfilaria have been implicated. Treatment involves keeping the horse in a darkened box, using atropine (intermittently to relax the iris and prevent adhesions), systemic and topical corticosteroids, and flunixin (Finadyne). Antibiotics may also be given, but are of dubious benefit.

The vitreous humour is seldom involved significantly in disease, but occasionally fragments of floating debris, possibly uveal in origin, may be seen in it, and have been blamed for horses shying and making startled movements for no apparent reason.

Retinal haemorrhage does occasionally occur in the horse, often leading to retinal detachment. Such haemorrhage may be due to periodic ophthalmia, to acute virus conditions such as influenza, or to anaphylactic conditions such as purpura. Detailed examination of the equine retina, and proper assessment of the significance of any changes seen therein are a matter, in most cases, for specialist help.

It is worth stressing that at the end of the day the most useful way of deciding the state of the horse's vision is to set up a series of tests involving stepping over poles laid on bricks, walking through a miniature bending course, moving among stones and bricks strewn irregularly on the ground, and so on. Reaction to light, to a moving finger, or a threatening finger, may all give useful information, provided the examiner's movement causes no tell-tale draught.

Finally it must be remembered, as discussed in the introduction, that this chapter is not intended to be exhaustive. Ophthalmology in the horse is a major study, and well beyond the scope of this very general chapter.

22 The heart

Clinical examination
Atrial fibrillation
   Partial heart block
   Complete heart block
   Cardiac palpitation
   Jugular distension
Cardiac hypertrophy
Chronic vegetative endocarditis
Pericarditis
Myocarditis
Congenital cardiac problems

The heart, like the eye, is an organ requiring sophisticated equipment and specialist knowledge, if a thorough and complete examination and assessment is to be carried out. In most companion animal practices with no specialist knowledge of equine cardiology, the aims, when considering a horse's heart, are to decide (a) whether there is any detectable abnormality and (b) whether any such abnormality is significant enough to necessitate the horse being rested from work, and a specialist cardiological opinion sought; or whether such abnormality poses no danger to horse or rider, and can therefore be noted and ignored.

It is vital to remember that one never examines a horse's heart in isolation; one examines the horse. The observations made during a general examination of the horse may be absolutely critical in attempting, later, to decide whether any cardiac abnormality is having a significant effect upon the horse's health and vigour.

Many horses suffer quite marked cardiac abnormalities for considerable periods without any discernible effect upon their well-being. The abnormality is often detected only during routine examination for health or insurance when, obviously, its significance is likely to be greatly exaggerated. It follows also that if such a horse suffers some coincidental illness during which cardiac auscultation is carried out as part of the clinical examination, then the cardiac abnormality is likely to be blamed for the animal's ill health. There is a much greater number of horses with cardiac abnormalities than of horses whose cardiac abnormalities are causing ill health, or are suggestive of danger. The differentiation is often a matter of commonsense assessment of all pertinent factors. The type of horse, its lifestyle, and the nature of the work demanded of it, must all be considered in the clinical assessment. There are many cardiac irregularities which would cause concern in a point-to-pointer or eventer which are of minor significance in a horse used only for occasional quiet hacking.

So the first requirement is a general clinical examination. Signs that might suggest possible cardiac pathology include discoloured mucous membranes, filling of superficial veins, jugular pulse, ascites, oedema, abducted elbows, dyspnoea particularly after slight exercise, cough, poor exercise tolerance, unsatisfactory performance, incoordination and collapse. Most of these signs may be found in diseases other than cardiac in origin: several of them occurring together give a better indication. In particular it is wise to beware of a story of unsatisfactory performance as the sole indication of cardiac disease, for a 'faulty heart' is almost universally blamed when a very expensive horse fails to live up to the owner's expectations. A jugular pulse is another trap for the unwary for many horses show an apparent jugular pulsation, and even a suggestion of jugular filling when the head and neck are below the horizontal position. These signs are due to the referred effect of the carotid pulse behind the jugular and the effect of gravity.

Even quite marked murmurs must be treated with suspicion, for many worm-infested, ill-fed and anaemic young horses show a gross systolic murmur, which disappears after good feeding and anthelmintic treatment.

It is wise, therefore, to be cautious about moving too quickly to a diagnosis of cardiac disease. Careful auscultation with an efficient stethoscope is still the most satisfactory method of assessing cardiac abnormality in the first instance. It is best to use an instrument with a flat disc and short tubes. Make sure that the ear pieces are not too tight, and practice whenever possible. Every opportunity should be taken of listening to the horse's heart even when the history and general picture do not necessarily suggest cardiac disease. Frequent practice is the only way to become proficient.

A number of factors may interfere with satisfactory use of the stethoscope. A thick and heavy coat, excessive fat on the chest wall, loud lung sounds, oesophageal sounds, colonic sounds and many extraneous environmental sounds may all make accurate auscultation difficult. It is important to find a quiet place, with no diversions to interfere with one's concentration. After examination of the heart at rest, it is essential to compare the picture with that after exercise. The exercise, however, should not be haphazard, but ought to be related to the work normally carried out by the patient. If fast work is expected of the horse it should be trotted for a few minutes, then re-examined; then cantered and re-examined; and finally galloped and re-examined. After the gallop the clinician should listen for some time, for immediately after galloping, the heart beat may be as high as 200 per minute, and it will be impossible to hear anything of significance until it slows considerably. The fitter the horse the sooner normal heart rate will be achieved, but although the initial decrease may be very rapid, the rate of decrease slows down considerably after the first few minutes and it may be an hour or more before completely normal rates are restored. It is important not to imagine a murmur when heart and respiratory rates have slowed to a point at which, for a short period, they are synchronous. At this stage the respiratory sound may sound very like a murmur. The same effect may occur in a horse in which the cardiac rate is fast enough for several beats to occur during each inspiration. There may be a slight movement of air in the adjacent lung, suggesting a murmur, with each heart beat, but these confusing sounds cease during expiration.

When first approaching a horse to listen to its heart, it is best to proceed quietly and slowly, avoiding sudden movement. If the horse is apprehensive the heart beat should be allowed to fall to a reasonably normal rate before making any assessment. The same rule applies when taking a horse's pulse rate; allow the pulse rate to slow down as much as possible before counting. The normal rate at rest varies in different horses from 36 to 42 per minute, but may be much slower in Thoroughbreds in training and in heavy draught horses. A pulse rate of from 28 to 32 per minute is not unusual in such animals. Such a slow rate in Thoroughbreds may lead to error in that when this type of animal is ill, and the pulse rate rises by 50% to, say, 45 per minute, the clinician does not realize that it is, in fact, significantly raised.

The anatomy of auscultation is as follows: the left ventricle is in contact with the chest wall from the third to the sixth rib on the left side. The apex beat can be heard in the lower third of the fifth intercostal space on the left side. This corresponds to a site just under the point of the left elbow. The area of auscultation on the left side can be extended by drawing the forelimb forwards. Two-thirds of the heart lies to the left of the midline, so that the right ventricle is close to, but not touching, the chest wall from the fourth to the sixth rib on the right side. Cardiac enlargement obviously pushes the heart nearer to the right side, and it becomes easier to hear it on that side.

Contraction of the ventricles and closure of the atrioventricular valves produces the sound traditionally described as 'lub'. This is systole. Diastole comprises ventricular relaxation and closure of the aortic and pulmonary valves giving the second sound 'dup'. Occasionally in fit horses with slow hearts one can hear a preliminary sound before the 'lub' sound, but this is neither constant nor important. A duplicated 'lub' sound is occasionally heard 'belub' due to asynchronization of the two sides of the heart, but it is far more common to hear a duplicated second or 'dup' sound due to uncoordinated closure of the aortic and pulmonary valves.

A murmur is a sound caused by turbulent blood movement

within the heart or adjacent great vessels. It is produced by damaged valves, septal defects or narrowing of the arteries. Systolic murmurs are those heard during contraction of the ventricles, and are usually caused by damaged atrioventricular valves, while diastolic murmurs are heard during relaxation of the ventricles, and are usually caused by damage to the aortic or pulmonary valves. Murmurs are often heard when hypertrophe of the heart has progressed to dilatation: in debilitating and anaemic conditions particularly in the young horse, in advanced chronic pulmonary disease and in severe arrhythmias.

The horse suffers from a group of cardiac arrhythmias. The most common of these is atrial fibrillation. The differentiation of the arrhythmias requires electrocardiographic examination, for all arrhythmias involve abnormalities in the conducting mechanisms of the heart, which are normally controlled by the sinoatrial node in the wall of the right atrium. Heart block occurs when the conducting mechanisms fail to control the coordination between the contractions of the atria and the contractions of the ventricles. In partial heart block ventricular contractions may be delayed, or some may be absent, i.e. the heart beat and pulse are irregular. All this is a matter for electrocardiographic study, but as a general rule if the missed beats occur regularly the problem is likely to be less significant than if the missed beats occur irregularly.

It is, however, vitally important that the missed beats do not occur during exercise – if normal cardiac rhythm re-appears during and for a while after exercise the prognosis is generally good, and many clinicians are satisfied if the heart at work is free of arrhythmias, whatever the position might be at rest.

Complete heart block occurs when the conducting mechanism between auricles and ventricles has failed completely: the ventricles then beat at their own intrinsic rate. In such cases the heart beat may be as little as 10–20 per minute, and is often irregular. Sometimes the ventricular beat is so slow, or in cases of partial heart block the interval between ventricular beats (i.e. the number of missed beats) is so large, even as many as seven in succession, that the horse faints and falls. The heart and pulse rate then improve, as they do on exercise, and transiently the horse regains normal rhythm. Notice that young, anaemic and frightened horses may show a loud, tumultuous and disorderly beating of the heart. This is cardiac palpitation, which usually occurs less often as the horse gets older and fitter, and need not give rise to concern.

A true jugular pulse in the horse (i.e. retrograde blood flow in the jugular vein) as opposed to the referred jugular pulsation previously described, is usually due to atrial fibrillation. Jugular distension may occur in several ways – it is generally part of the cycle of chronic venous congestion which includes oedema and which may start in the heart, lungs or even the liver. It may start as a local valvular lesion – usually the right atrioventricular valve. In atrial fibrillation the degree of jugular filling may correspond to the duration of the diastole – if diastole is long the jugular distends.

It should be re-emphasized that a dropped beat in a fit horse after a period of rest should not be regarded as a pathological arrhythmia if the dropped beat is restored on exercise, the pulse is of normal type and volume, and exercise tolerance is acceptable. A significant arrhythmia is usually irregular, with dyspnoea on exertion, even to the point of collapse. The pulse at rest is irregular in rate and rhythm.

Cardiac hypertrophe in the horse is by no means unusual. It occurs whenever the heart is consistently heavily or abnormally worked, provided that the heart muscle can compensate. But if the stress becomes too severe, or occurs too quickly for muscular compensation to occur, then cardiac dilatation supervenes, as in advanced chronic pulmonary disease. The majority of race-horses in training, if properly fed and exercised, develop some hypertrophe of the heart. The area of cardiac dullness increases, the pulse becomes slow and full, and the horse develops increased exercise tolerance. Dilatation, however, usually causes a severe systolic murmur and an irregularly beating heart.

Chronic vegetative endocarditis occurs occasionally in the horse. The vegetative lesions usually affect the atrioventricular valves, particularly on the right. The vegetation may start as an allergic reaction, but is usually bacterial. Streptococci are particularly involved. Clinical signs include weight loss, fever, anorexia, shifting joint lameness, markedly raised pulse rate, anaemia, leucocytosis, neutrophilia, with cardiac murmurs, usually right sided and systolic. Eventually congestive heart failure occurs. There may be pulmonary oedema and dyspnoea in left-sided cases, or ascites and liver enlargement in right-sided syndromes.

Pericarditis may follow viral conditions such as influenza, may be secondary to some types of pneumonia and pleurisy, or may occasionally be traumatic following penetration of the oesophagus by a foreign body which reaches the pericardium. The clinical signs start with pyrexia and thoracic pain. Friction rubs may be detected on auscultation. Then fluid collects in the pericardial sac and fluid splashing and tinkling occur. The pulse rate becomes fast and often irregular. Murmurs and arrhythmias usually occur. Congestive heart failure and circulatory collapse eventually follow. Sudden death may result, either from very severe arrhythmia, or from pericardial rupture and fatal haemorrhage.

Myocarditis develops from a variety of causes, usually infective. It may occur by local spread from the pericardium, as in tuberculosis. It may be streptococcal following strangles or influenza. Occasionally aberrant strongyle damage is involved. Endocardial lesions may spread to the myocardium. Haemorrhagic and degenerative changes may occur in purpura, or even in severe anaemia. Clinical signs include raised temperature and pulse rate, inappetence, exercise intolerance and dyspnoea, general venous congestion, circulatory collapse, and death from heart failure or even from rupture of one of the chambers of the heart.

Congenital cardiac problems do occasionally occur in the foal and include:

- Patent ductus arteriosis
- Persistent foramen ovale
- Interventricular septal defects
- Tetralogy of Fallot

Sudden death occurs occasionally in fast working horses as a result of rupture of one of the great vessels within the chest.

23 Diseases of the foal

Neonatal infections
    Sleepy foal disease (actinobacillus; shigella)
    Coliform septicaemias and diarrhoea
    Streptococcal septicaemias and joint-ill
    Staphylococcal organisms
    Klebsiella
Diarrhoea
    Neonatal infections
    Rotavirus
    Salmonella
    Clostridia
    Corynebacterium equi
    Parasites
    Oestral diarrhoea
Respiratory conditions
    Complications of the neonatal
       pyosepticaemias
    Ascariasis
    C. equi
    Fractured ribs and bruised heart
    Equine herpes virus 2
Neurological conditions
    Prematurity/dysmaturity
    Viral ataxia (EHV1)
    Neonatal maladjustment syndromes

'Colic' syndromes
    Tympanitic colic
    Volvulus
    Intussusception
    Retained meconium
    Ruptured bladder
    Strongylosis
Orthopaedic conditions
Haemolytic disease
Hepatitis (Tyzzer's)
Tetanus
Steatitis, polymyositis, hyperlipaemia
Congenital conditions

For an introductory text to diseases of the foal, refer to *Equine Stud Farm Medicine* (Rossdale and Ricketts, 1980).

Full-term gestation takes approximately 340 days. Foals born at between 300 and 320 days are classified as premature or immature. The causes are vague, but include stress often linked with placental malfunction. These foals are born weak, take a long while to stand, and have a poor suck reflex. A normal foal should be on its feet well within 2 hours. Premature foals tend to show low-grade abdominal pain after feeding. The skin is soft, silky, and develops bedsores very easily; the hooves may be very soft.

A dysmature foal is one born after 320 days' pregnancy, but which still looks immature. Such a foal almost certainly suffered placental difficulties. On the other hand it is not unusual for foals to be born up to 1 month, and even 2 months, late, and yet be perfectly normal. They are much better late than early. Foals which are born early as a result of equine herpes virus 1 (EHV1) infection in the mare, in effect abortion cases, are often weak, jaundiced, and unable to stand or suckle. They may well not survive.

Immediate intake of an adequate volume of colostrum of the relevant composition is vital to the newborn. One litre in the first 6 hours is a must. It has been said that a foal, born normal from a normal placenta, will not suffer, and certainly will not die from neonatal infections, if it has received sufficient colostrum in the first 6 hours of life. This is probably largely true. There are, however, a number of factors which may affect a foal's normality at this critical time. The placenta may have been abnormal or inadequate. There may have been placentitis. The mare may have developed laminitis: there may have been dystokia, prolonged labour, or even caesarean section. Or the mare may have been infected by EHV1. The foal may be premature, or dysmature, or anatomically abnormal, e.g. contracted tendons. All these factors and others increase the foal's susceptibility to neonatal disease.

We must remember that when newborn foals are ill they tend not to show clear-cut differential symptoms. They just look like sick foals, and most sick foals look alike. The reaction to disease stimulus is blurred in the newborn, and so may be response to treatment. Diagnosis may be difficult: it is vital to carry out clinical and laboratory examination very early, and from the therapeutic point of view it is wise to play safe and cover the possibilities.

It is therefore better to work, initially, in wider and more general differential groups:

(1) *Infective conditions,* which all to some extent show a raised temperature, lethargy even to the point of sleepiness, a reduced strength of suck, and leucocytosis. Infective conditions in the foal may well be pyosepticaemic, but the primary sites of infection include gut, joints, liver, kidney, brain and lungs. Among the conditions are sleepy foal disease (*Actinobacillus equuli*), coliform septicaemias and diarrhoea, joint-ill (streptococci/staphylococci), klebsiella conditions and EHV1.

(2) *Non-infective conditions* include:

    (a) *Gross behavioural disturbances,* e.g. neonatal maladjustment syndrome (NMS) (barkers, wanderers, dummies, convulsives).

    (b) *Anatomical abnormalities,* e.g. contracted tendons: pervious urachus.

    (c) *Mechanical conditions,* e.g. retention of meconium.

    (d) *Fetal/maternal immune reactions* – haemolytic disease.

Now we should consider foal diseases in more detail.

Infective conditions in the neonatal period

'Sleepy foal' disease – (*Actinobacillus equuli*, shigella)

This condition is less common than previously, probably as a result of the widespread use of prophylactic antibiotics in the newborn foal. The organism may be present in uterus and vagina, also in the mouth and nasal passages of the mare. Clinical disease occurs within the first few days of life, usually at 48 hours. The usual picture is of a sleepy flaccid foal which will not suck. Temperature may be raised at first, but becomes subnormal. Death may occur in the septicaemic phase, but if the foal lives a little longer diarrhoea and dehydration may develop, as may uraemic convulsions. The urine is high in urea and contains much debris. A little later, if the foal survives, swellings of joints and tendon sheaths occur. There is marked leucocytosis. If death occurs in the first 24–36 hours of life there are unlikely to be significant lesions. In later deaths there will be microabscesses in the kidney cortex, plus changes in the joint capsules and tendon sheaths, varying from congestion and excess synovial fluid to purulent arthritis and taenosynovitis. The organism may be isolated from the joints, kidney abscesses, or even the urine.

Coliform septicaemias and diarrhoea

These are steadily increasing in importance, in line with the increasing concentration and crowding of foals. There are usually stress factors involved, a similar story to that of other species. The disease appears from 2 to 28 days – the younger the foal the more tendency towards septicaemia; older foals are more likely to be diarrhoeic. Purulent ascites, purulent arthritic changes, septic pleurisy and peritonitis may also develop. Many cases of coliform disease show congestion of mucous membranes with a definite jaundice. It is very important that this jaundice does not lead to a mistaken diagnosis of haemolytic disease. The membranes in haemolytic disease, however, will be pale and jaundiced as opposed to congested and jaundiced, while the packed cell volume (PCV) will be greatly lowered rather than considerably raised.

Streptococcal septicaemias and joint-ill

These are less common than the coliform infections. In the very young an acute septicaemic picture with collapse may occur; joint-ill and navel-ill appear in older animals with raised temperature and lameness. The latter form is more common.

Staphylococcal and klebsiella organisms producing pyosepticaemia

When dealing with valuable foals showing severe neonatal disease, the vagueness of the differential picture suggests that full haematological and biochemical parameters should be used to confirm, or otherwise, the clinical estimation. Infected foals may well show haemoconcentration, leucocytosis, hypogly-caemia, positive blood cultures, raised blood urea and raised globulins. It is vital that dehydration and electrolyte loss be quickly monitored and corrected.

In the field, however, it is necessary to look at disease from a much wider viewpoint, and work out a differential diagnostic approach to the main presenting symptoms.

Diarrhoea

Diarrhoea occurs in foals from a day or two old up to the age of six months, which is usually regarded as the theoretical end limit of foalhood. There are many causes. It may develop during the course of a neonatal pyosepticaemia, e.g. *A. equulis* and particularly coliform. Coliforms and klebsiella can occur as primarily enteric conditions in older foals several weeks of age, without septicaemic changes, whilst rotavirus and salmonella (particularly *S. typhimurium*) may be very important in diarrhoeic conditions in still older foals up to several months old. Rotaviral diarrhoea is watery with a greenish tinge. Temperature may be 105°F (40.5°C) at first, but drops as diarrhoea continues and dehydration occurs. Leucocytosis and neutrophilia may occur. Salmonella and rotavirus may occur in the same foal – the salmonella probably being secondary, and certainly much more dangerous than the rotavirus. It can kill young foals very quickly, the initial high temperatures dropping to subnormal while the scour and dehydration worsen to the point of collapse. Older foals may merely show a subacute picture with chronic diarrhoea. Occasionally a foal may recover from rotavirus infection to the extent that it appears perfectly well, but continues to pass sloppy unformed faeces for as much as a year. Rotavirus is becoming steadily more important, and is beginning to appear even in the neonatal phase. Confirmatory diagnosis is by ELISA or fluorescent antibody tests, electron microscopy, and virus culture. *Campylobacter* species may also cause diarrhoea in foals from 2 to 4 months of age (approximately).

Clostridia can cause very serious and usually fatal disease in foals. *Cl. perfringens (welchii)* type B (the organism of lamb dysentery) and *Cl. difficile* are the organisms involved. There is an initial high temperature falling rapidly; abdominal pain is followed by severe diarrhoea and great depression. The faeces may contain blood. Post-mortem lesions include severe congestion, discolouration, ulceration and necrosis of the gut. It is possible, though difficult, to demonstrate clostridial toxins in the gut content. If the disease is suspected it may help to give in-contact lamb dysentery serum to counteract *Cl. perfringens* type B.

Corynebacterium equi, primarily a respiratory invader, may show a secondary diarrhoea.

Prominent in the aetiology of diarrhoea in the older foal are *parasites*. Ascaris may produce sufficient gut irritation to set up diarrhoea, but is much more important in the lungs. *Strongylus vulgaris* larvae complete their cycle between 5 and 6 months, and if ingested in the first few days of life may cause anaemia and diarrhoea from 6 months of age onwards following their return to the gut. There may already have been interference with growth, a pot-belly, anaemia and intermittent abdominal pain from some 2 months old onwards during the transabdominal migration along the vessels of the anterior mesenteric tree, and back to the gut. During this migratory period, and until the larvae are back in the gut again, there is more likely to be constipation than diarrhoea. Probably the most important parasite during the foal's early life is *Strongyloides westeri*. Crowded studs, insanitary conditions, and foals in suboptimal health lead to heavy infestation with this parasite, causing profuse diarrhoea, dehydration, and weight loss usually at 2–3 months of age.

So-called *oestral diarrhoea* should also be remembered. This relatively benign diarrhoea occurs when the foal is 9–10 days old and the dam comes into oestrus. It may also occur at the next oestrus some 3 weeks later. It may be due to changes in milk composition while the mare is in heat, but it is at least as likely that the foal is neglected and stressed at this time, particularly if the mare and foal have to travel long distances to the stallion.

In spite of the varied aetiology of diarrhoea in the foal it is very true that whatever specific treatment is used, the important part of the therapy is the replacement of fluid and electrolytes including sodium, potassium and chloride, also glucose and bicarbonate, given orally or intravenously depending on the condition of the foal.

Respiratory conditions

Complications of the neonatal pyosepticaemias

Ascariasis – the 'thumps'

The effects of the migration through the lungs of ascarid larvae, which cause rapid forceful respirations with a clear-cut jerk or 'thump' at the end of each respiration. There may be loss of weight, but on the whole minimal permanent damage is done.

Corynebacterium equi

This causes pyaemia and pneumonia in foals aged 2 months plus. These foals usually spend several weeks in a vague non-thriving condition, before they deteriorate suddenly with acute pneumonia. There are large abscesses in the lungs and occasionally in the mesenteric nodes. There is sometimes diarrhoea. Patients may remain chronically ill for a considerable time.

Fractured ribs and bruised heart

This syndrome occurs during parturition as a result of rough and hasty forced traction by the attendants. The ribs on the left side fracture at the costochondral junctions over the heart. Overriding of the ends causes impingement of the pleura and pericardium and damage to the heart. Sudden death, or an acute respiratory picture may occur.

Equine herpes virus 2

This virus affects unweaned foals several months old, causing a chronic nasal discharge and cough.

Neurological conditions

Prematurity and dysmaturity

These conditions have already been mentioned on p. 153.

Viral ataxia (EHV1)

EHV1 infecting the dam is passed to the fetus causing nerve damage and ataxia.

Neonatal maladjustment syndromes (NMS)

These syndromes are very important and comprise *barkers, wanderers, dummies* and *convulsives.*

These cases are born normally to term, but within a few hours they show behavioural disturbances. There is almost complete loss of the suck reflex, and the foal cannot recognize the mare. Blindness and nervous signs of a convulsive type appear. There is respiratory overactivity. The syndrome is possibly due to partial asphyxia at birth. It occurs in acute and chronic forms – the acute form is known as the 'barker' foal. It shows acute central nervous symptoms, galloping in incoordinate fashion around the box, running blindly into the walls, falling over backwards, making spasmodic leaps, sweating, blowing, and making loud fox-like barking noises, while gasping for breath due to atelectasis and cerebral anoxia. The prognosis is grave, although the foal which has been on its feet and suckling well before the attack has a better chance.

After the acute attack the foal is exhausted and temporarily blind. It cannot suck, nor can it find the teat. Swallowing is difficult. When it is on its feet it wanders aimlessly, hence the description 'wanderer'. A foal may become a wanderer without having suffered an acute attack.

'Colic' syndromes

Flatulent or tympanitic colic

This is occasionally seen in quite young foals. The pain is acute, and the violent behaviour of the 'patient' may be mistaken for fits.

Volvulus

Volvulus may occur as a complication of tympany. It usually affects the posterior ileum.

Intussusception

This occurs occasionally. The foal is in continual acute pain. It walks backwards, lies on its back, rolls, sweats and literally throws itself about. It becomes toxic fairly quickly, and an early decision is important. Surgery is advisable if pain continues for more than 1 hour, or before that if the pain is less acute, but the foal looks worse.

Retained meconium

Meconium retention is common, particularly in colt foals in the first 36 hours of life. The impaction is in the last foot or so of the gut, usually in the last few inches of the rectum. The foal crouches and strains with its tail upwards, and often walks backwards.

Ruptured bladder

Ruptured bladder is often seen in colt foals following retained meconium, so that one must differentiate between retained meconium, ruptured bladder, and retained meconium plus ruptured bladder. Signs appear from 2 or 3 days old, up to 7 days or so. The foal becomes dull, obviously uncomfortable, and does not suck. It tries to pass urine, and often some comes. The foal again may strain and walk backwards. The tear in the bladder is generally along the dorsal surface.

Strongyle invasion of the abdomen

This may cause ill thrift, anaemia, and episodes of abdominal pain or discomfort, often with constipation and pot-belly, at any time from 8 weeks or so onwards.

Orthopaedic conditions

In the foal orthopaedic conditions include:

(1) Joint-ill resulting from streptococcal infection.
(2) Complications of the neonatal pyosepticaemias.
(3) Congenital conditions including contracted or extended tendons.
(4) Trauma – very common in the young foal which seems particularly prone to environmental injury.

Haemolytic disease of the newborn foal

This condition occurs in Thoroughbred foals almost exclusively, and is a disease of isoimmunization. The incidence of the disease is not accurately known, but it is certainly rare. It is analogous to the rhesus factor condition in the human, but the horse has a very complicated blood grouping system, including not one but at least seven antigenic factors attached to the red cells and corresponding to the human rhesus factor. For the disease to occur we need:

(1) A sire with the blood antigen and a dam without.
(2) A fetus which has inherited the sire's antigen.
(3) The mare must become sensitized during pregnancy, possibly by leakage of fetal red cells through defects, haemorrhages, or necrotic areas in the placental structure into the maternal circulation.
(4) The newborn foal must suck, for there is no placental antibody transfer in the equine species.

It is unusual for the mare to produce a haemolytic first foal. She usually requires several matings to the same sire, or a sire with similar red cell antigenic structure, before a damaging antibody level builds up. This is always likely in concentrated breeding areas such as Newmarket. The disease may occur with a first foal if there have been previous abortions to sires with similar antigens.

Clinical symptoms vary in intensity according to the antibody involved. Very acute cases may produce symptoms within some hours of birth. The foal may be lethargic and sleepy, lying down a lot, usually on its sternum, with its chin on the ground. It may yawn excessively. Then haemoglobinuria occurs with pale mucous membranes which rapidly become jaundiced. Respirations become rapid and panting in nature. Faeces tend to be very yellow, but are constipated rather than diarrhoeic. Eventually the foal is unable to stand, its temperature becomes subnormal, its pulse rate very fast, with a loudly thumping heart easily audible to persons nearby. At the other end of the scale are foals where signs do not appear until several days of age, and may amount to nothing more than lethargy and mild jaundice, seen best in conjunctival membranes.

Differential diagnosis is important, for early treatment of severe cases is all important. Obviously it includes all the infective septicaemic conditions of the newborn, but these are likely to show a raised temperature *early* in the disease, although it may fall later. Mucous membranes are usually dirty and congested, rather than the clear yellow colour of uncomplicated jaundice, though a coliform septicaemia may cause a rather dirty jaundiced appearance. PCV will always be normal or raised in the infective conditions, but significantly lowered in iso-immunization cases. Another cause of a clear yellow jaundice is physiological icterus of the newborn, but these foals are not ill and have normal PCV levels. It is also worth noting that a foal with retained meconium of several days standing may become jaundiced. It is, however, usually standing uncomfortably rather than lying and lethargic. Basically the PCV is the key – haemolytic disease cannot be present with a normal or raised PCV, it will be considerably lowered.

Hepatitis (Tyzzer's disease)

This disease is caused by *Bacillus piliformis*, a spore-bearing bacillus which causes acute hepatitis between 2 and 6 weeks of age as a result of ingestion of spores from equine faeces. The foal may be found dead, or shows great depression and collapse. There may be fever and jaundice. These signs are rapidly followed by collapse, coma and death. Post-mortem examination shows a grossly enlarged liver with areas of necrosis surrounded by inflammatory change.

Tetanus

Tetanus is always a possibility in a young foal, unless the mare is fully vaccinated and boosted prior to parturition. The site of entry is probably the umbilicus in most cases.

Steatitis, polymyositis and hyperlipaemia

Hyperlipaemia

Hyperlipaemia is usually seen in older foals, from the age of 5 months upwards. They are usually foals of the small breeds, Shetland and Welsh foals are particularly susceptible, and they are usually overfat. The condition occurs when there is sudden dietary setback, producing an energy deficit. Coincidental illness, heavy snowfall, deliberate dieting in an effort by the owner to reduce the foal's weight quickly, may all be involved. The liver shows massive fatty change, whilst the blood plasma becomes so fatty that the blood settles out in a collecting tube looking like a blood clot in a tube full of cream. The foal is very dull and lethargic, and stands very still. There may be a scanty greasy diarrhoea in some cases. The condition is accompanied by a myopathy of the masseter and related muscles to cause the so called maxillary myositis. The foal cannot use its lips, nor can it swallow properly: food and water run back out of the mouth during attempts to swallow.

Polymyositis

Polymyositis may affect poor, ill-thrifty, and deprived foals on marginal land, especially in the winter months. Some authorities suggest that there is a predisposing vitamin E/selenium deficiency. The condition, also known as *nutritional myopathy*, *rhabdomyolysis* or *muscular dystrophy*, is triggered off by exercise –

any combination of muscles or all muscles, may be affected. There is suddenly developing stiffness in many muscle groups, causing great pain, sweating and respiratory distress. The foal chokes on food in its pharynx, because the oesophageal muscle is non-functional and the oesophagus is packed with food material. There is often myocardial damage: there is dark red myoglobin in the urine. Breathing becomes more and more distressed; standing becomes difficult, the foal sways, staggers, and collapses struggling on the ground. Death follows recumbency without great delay. There is sometimes an accompanying hyperlipaemia. Creatine phosphokinase (CPK) and aspartate aminotransferase (AAT) are very high indeed.

Differential diagnosis includes the various forms of acute colic, hypocalcaemia and hypomagnesaemia. *Steatitis* (yellow fat disease, fat necrosis) is seen in Highland foals, and occasionally in Shetlands, sometimes associated with *muscular dystrophy*. it affects the crest, the omental and abdominal fat, and much of the subcutaneous fat. Affected fat is hard, necrotic, and may contain pools of degenerate fatty liquid within the hard mass. In the subcutaneous areas this gives the appearance of multiple abscesses. Sometimes the affected areas are fairly localized, but often most of the body fat is affected and the foal may look dull and depressed with a raised temperature and episodes of pain, believed to be due to the pressure of hard, coagulated and necrotic fat in the omentum and mesentery. Steatitis, like muscular dystrophy, is believed in some quarters to be associated with vitamin E metabolism. Some affected foals may develop hyperlipaemia.

Congenital conditions of the foal

A large number of congenital conditions appear in the foal. The more important are:

Entropion (see Chapter 21)

In the foal entropion is relatively benign, and may correct itself within the first few weeks of life. To prevent corneal damage until this happens regular manual eversion may work, or two folds of skin may be sutured together beneath the eye, but in some cases more radical surgical interference can be necessary to reduce the condition.

Guttural pouch tympany

Due to faulty functioning of the distal end of the Eustachian tube. The pouch takes in air during normal pharyngeal movement. The condition may be unilateral or bilateral.

Atresia ani or coli

Atresia coli is obviously much more serious.

Scrotal/inguinal hernia

In the foal the hernial sac may be very large at birth, but tends to appear progressively smaller as time goes on.

Pervious urachus

This is often missed, for there is no urine trickle from the urachus, and the bulk of the urine formed may be passed normally. A wet smelly patch, however, forms on the ventral abdomen, predisposing to cystitis. As long as the skin and hair are kept clean, the urachus usually closes within 14 days.

Cardiac septal defects

When these occur they lead to steadily increasing exercise intolerance as the foal gets older and takes more and more exercise. Dyspnoea and discoloured mucous membranes occur on exertion. The foal may collapse while exercising. Massive cardiac murmurs are heard.

Contracted flexor tendons

Contracted flexor tendons of both forelegs are not uncommon. Provided that the weight of the foal tends to press the foot backwards and downwards onto the sole rather than forward and downward onto the front wall, the foal will recover without treatment, otherwise stretching, splinting or surgery of varying severity will be required.

Umbilical hernia

This is usually noticed first when the foal is several weeks old. This type of hernia is generally harmless in the horse, containing omental tissue only. By the time the foal is 6 months old the hernia is often only just noticeable. Diagnosis is generally easy, for the sac is easily reducible, and there is no pain, heat nor inflammatory swelling. Differential diagnosis involves umbilical abscess which is hard, often painful on pressure, and inflamed. It cannot, of course, be reduced, and after a varying period it shows a fluctuating area. In time the whole of the superficial (ventral) border of the abscess fluctuates and becomes cool and relatively non-painful. It is particularly at this stage that mistakes occur. It is vital, however sure the clinician may be that he is dealing with an abscess, that he carries out an exploratory needle puncture before committing himself to surgical incision. It must also be remembered that hernias sometimes develop at the base of a longstanding umbilical abscess as a result of damage to the ventral abdominal wall from the infection. Umbilical abscesses must always be opened with care, and the base of the abscess cavity searched with the fingers for any sign of a hernial sac before the foal is released.

Combined immunodeficiency (CID)

This condition is found in Arab foals. These foals are unable to develop antibodies, and produce no resistance to viruses or bacteria, particularly adenovirus. Repeated infections occur due to adenovirus, and also to cryptosporidia, coliforms and staphylococci. Eventually death occurs. It seems that both sire and dam must be CID carriers before the clinical condition occurs in the foal.

Diagnosis depends on finding less than 1000 lymphocytes per mm^3 in the foal's blood; a lack of immunoglobulin M (IgM) production by the foal; and at post-mortem examination hypoplasia of the lymphoreticular system.

Cerebellar hypoplasia

An ataxic condition involving serious incoordination and falling from birth onwards.

Myelopathy of the cervical vertebral canal – the wobbler syndrome

A very important condition which is present at birth, but is often not noticed until the foal is handled for breaking and schooling.

It often seems to become more noticeable after the youngster (if male) has been cast for castration. The condition is a congenital deformity of the cervical spine, occurring in the midcervical region, and resulting in the distortion of the vertebral canal at that point. The symptoms include hindquarter incoordination and swaying. There is an ataxic hindleg action with defective foot placement. Sometimes the forelegs are also affected to some extent. The young horse finds it difficult to back or to turn, and easily falls. Confirmation is by lateral radiography of the neck.

Reference

Rossdale, P. D. and Ricketts, S. W. (1980) *Equine Stud Farm Medicine,* 2nd edn, Baillière Tindall, London, pp. 277–421

24 The laboratory

Indications for haematology and blood biochemistry and interpretation of results

Increasingly, over the past 15–20 years, it has become customary for the equine clinician to back up his clinical examination by frequent recourse to the laboratory. Laboratory work has become not only fashionable but very expensive. More and more laboratories compete to offer a wider and wider range of tests, and more and more equine practices set up their own laboratories to speed up the results and to obtain a share of the financial return.

Why has this trend become so important, so rapidly?

(1) Equine internal medicine may present difficult clinical problems. A number of common syndromes, e.g. chronic weight loss, chronic colic, chronic diarrhoea and poor performance, have multiple and varied aetiologies in which the laboratory may be very helpful.
(2) Blood and other samples can gain you valuable time in obscure cases.
(3) Laboratory results may convince the client that you are talking sense. He or she may disbelieve you, but will always believe the laboratory. But you must make sure you get the right results and interpret them correctly.
(4) Horse clients are, by and large, knowledgeable and competitive, have become interested in laboratory work, and may well feel dissatisfied if you do not take samples as part of your examination.

But, laboratory diagnosis has many pitfalls:

Laboratory results are only valid when related to the clinical picture. *Only the clinician is competent to carry out this assessment.* If the laboratory results do not make sense when considered against the clinical picture, then they should be regarded with suspicion, *for the horse is always right.*

Over the past decade, we have all come to realize the importance of the laboratory in the medicine of the horse, but some of us have become laboratory fanatics. BEWARE. One can get to the stage at which, when presented with a sick horse, one descends upon it with a variety of bottles and needles and rushes off to the laboratory with many samples. It is not until all the tests have produced negative results that one returns to look at the horse and realize that it has pus in the foot! which we should have seen in the first place if we had looked.

This habit of sending for every known parameter in the hope that among them will be the right answer is quite unforgiveable. The clinician should select the laboratory tests most likely to help by confirming or refuting the diagnostic ideas forming as he examines the animal – *he should be the master, and not the slave, of laboratory procedures.*

Remember that the book normal range for any test carried out in the horse is very wide and of limited use diagnostically, for the horse is not one animal as far as laboratory parameters are concerned, but several. So:

- There is a normal range for the horse.
- There is a normal range for ponies, one for Thoroughbreds and another for heavy horses.
- There is a normal range for Thoroughbreds at rest and another for Thoroughbreds in training.
- There is a normal range for foals and another for adult horses.

So, any laboratory result has to be interpreted in relation to the breed, age and work pattern of the horse concerned.

There is also a normal range for each individual. For example, how often has one examined a horse with a white cell count of 9000 mm^3 and regarded it as normal, only to find when recovery occurs that this horse's normal white cell count is 5000.

Notice too that results can vary quite widely in one quite normal horse, from day to day. One series of results can be most misleading – one needs serial results day by day for several days, and this is prohibitively expensive.

Laboratory results are often misleading for a number of reasons:

(1) To do with the horse – e.g.
- *Young horses* have high SAP (serum alkaline phosphatase) figures; horses at work may have high SCPK (serum creatine phosphokinase) and high SGOT (serum aspartate aminotransferase) levels.
- Fit horses have high RBC (red blood cell) counts, while stressed horses have high white cell counts.
Fear, flight, and fight alter many things.
(2) To do with the clinician – e.g. be quiet. Don't bustle the horse. Don't frighten him. Perfect your intravenous technique. Don't take bloods immediately after exercise. A 2-hour rest is optimal. Get the bloods into the laboratory quickly – many

results will be inaccurate after 24 hours in transit, e.g. CPK will drop markedly and SDH be quite inaccurate in 24 hours. White cell figures are hopelessly affected in 24 hours, especially in warm temperatures, or if the sample is shaken.

(3) *To do with the laboratory.* Different laboratories perform the serum enzyme tests at different temperatures, e.g. 25°C, 30°C or 37°C. Results differ depending upon temperature: 25°C gives narrower and tighter result patterns but most laboratories work at 30°C or 37°C. 30°C is fairly good to the clinician, but 37°C, the preferred temperature of · many laboratories, gives a very wide normal range more difficult to interpret, until one becomes very familiar with the results obtained.

Laboratories use different methods, find a laboratory you like, and then stick to it. Use their normal range figures; keep in touch with them; take the samples properly; use the right preservatives; get the samples quickly to the laboratory, and provide a good history.

If your mind works in units which differ from the laboratory's, then get a good conversion table.

Do not regard the technician as infallible. Even technicians make mistakes, e.g. putting the decimal point in the wrong place, misreading your request form, etc.

So, we need a tidy routine laboratory procedure which will confirm or refute, as far as possible, the more important aetiological factors for the conditions which provide us with diagnostic difficulty in the horse. We need a minimum number of tests and each test must be directly related to a specific disease lesion, and must be reliable and cheap.

Thus, we need to know the disease syndromes most likely to need laboratory assessment. Obviously, many diseases do not require laboratory tests at all. However, some syndromes have a wide differential diagnosis, which may be clinically obscure. Fortunately, they form a pattern, i.e. the same group of tests will give the answer provided it is rigidly adhered to.

Disease syndromes include:

(A) Acute syndromes

(1) *Colics* – in which we need to know whether we are dealing with an *abdominal crisis*, or not, i.e. to measure haemoconcentration, toxaemia, acidosis and shock. So, we need PCV as a guide to haemoconcentration; urea and chloride as a

guide to toxaemia and electrolyte loss; pH and lactate (30 mg/100 ml) as a guide to acidosis. The laboratory here is prognostic, not diagnostic.

(B) Chronic syndromes
(1) Chronic colics, i.e. low-grade abdominal pain with weight loss.
(2) Chronic weight loss, with or without *pain,* with or without diarrhoea.
(3) Dull anorexic lethargic horses, e.g. acute and chronic liver and kidney disease.
(4) Horses showing poor performance, e.g. anaemic horses.
(5) Stiff horses, e.g. muscular lesions, brucellosis, azoturia, etc.

So we need a simple metabolic profile which will cover liver, gut, kidney, muscle and general anaemic conditions.

Take:

- A sequestrene (EDTA) blood.
- 20 ml clotted or heparinized blood (according to your laboratory's preference).
- A faeces sample.

The routine laboratory scan of such a case includes:

(1) Examination of an EDTA (sequestrene) sample for the red and white blood cell picture:
   (a) The red cell picture – Remember the wide range of normals depending upon breed, type and workload of the horse. See haematology data below.

   Be particularly careful not to frighten the horse, nor to produce violent evasive movement, for fright and exercise lift the packed cell volume (PCV) markedly. In fact, if the PCV does not rise by 10–15% after moderate exercise, there is probably something wrong.

   The PCV helps to assess dehydration and anaemia. But beware of the horse that is both anaemic and dehydrated – the PCV may appear to be normal! For full assessment of the red cell picture, you also need the haemoglobin (Hb) level and the red cell count, and preferably the mean corpuscular volume (MCV) and the mean corpuscular haemoglobin concentration (MCHC) as well.

Anaemic red cell pictures appear in:
- Starvation and debilitating disease.
- Chronic liver damage.
- Chronic·blood loss – often parasitic.
- Neoplasia, e.g. lymphosarcoma.
- Folic acid deficiencies – not uncommon in stabled horses in late winter receiving poor hay and no grass.
- Iron deficiency – rare except after chronic blood loss, e.g. parasitism.
- Postviral anaemia – a very real problem in Thoroughbreds after viral respiratory conditions.

The type of anaemia may be useful, e.g. normochromic normocytic initially in blood loss; macrocytic in folic acid deficiency; microcytic in iron deficiency.

The red cell picture is always a useful guide to the training progress of a Thoroughbred, and the rise after exercise may help to assess the state of fitness.

(b) *The white cell picture* is not as useful as is generally believed.

A rise in the *total count* indicates infection, and/or stress. But beware – there is much variation. The white cell count needs to be 15 000 plus per mm^3, before any deductions can be made regarding bacterial infection. *Notice* also that the total count may be very high (15 000–20 000 per mm^3) in severe migratory strongyle damage, and may easily reach 20 000 per mm^3 in lymphosarcomatous invasion. Contrary to expectations, this figure will probably be made up largely of polymorphs. Massive lymphocyte counts are normally seen only in bone marrow involvement and some cases of widespread lymph node invasion.

Viral infections tend to lower the total white cell count with a disproportionate rise in the lymphocyte and monocyte percentages, whilst the early stages of very acute and septicaemic bacterial infections such as salmonellosis may show a very low (1000–2000 per mm^3) total white cell count.

Band forms are rarely raised in horses except in very acute infections. Because there is so much variation in the total white cell count and the polymorph and lymphocyte percentages, it is much safer to convert the percentages to absolute figures, which allow more realistic interpretation.

Raised eosinophil levels may suggest allergies or parasitic infestations, but allergies and parasitic infestations do not necessarily produce eosinophilia. Raised monocyte levels may, or may not, indicate virus infections or tuberculosis. The significance of basophilia is very doubtful, though many haematologists regard it as a grave prognostic sign.

Haematological data

Normal range (Thoroughbreds)

Haemoglobin	14–19 g/100 ml
Red cells	$7.5–11 \times 10^6/mm^3$
PCV (haematocrit)	36–52% – average 40% PCV
MCV	38–55 fl
MCHC	32–38%
Leucocytes	5000–9000 per mm^3
Eosinophils	0–350 per mm^3
Neutrophils	Bands 0–500 per mm^3
	Adults 2000–6000 per mm^3
Basophils	0–100 per mm^3
Lymphocytes	2000–4000 per mm^3
Monocytes	0–500 per mm^3

Hill ponies (alright above)

Haemoglobin	11.0 g/100 ml
Red cells	$6.5 \times 10^6/mm^3$
Haematocrit	30%

Thoroughbreds (anaemic below)

Haemoglobin	12 g/100 ml
Red cells	$7 \times 10^6/mm^3$
Haematocrit	should be at least 38% in working Thoroughbred

(2) *Examination of a clotted or heparinized blood (according to the preference of the laboratory) for:*
(a) *Blood urea*
- Raised in cases of urinary obstruction
- Raised in many cases of kidney disease
- Usually high in chronic grass sickness
- May be raised in any case associated with rapid loss of flesh

If the blood urea is high, urine analysis should be carried out, as this may confirm kidney damage.

(b) *Sorbitol dehydrogenase (SDH) and gamma glutamyl trans-ferase (GGT).* These are cellular enzymes whose concentration in the serum rises when large number of cells are disrupted or degenerate. *SDH* is very useful for it is present mainly in the liver of the horse and so is reasonably specific for liver damage. It gives a measurement of acute liver damage, rising rapidly at the onset of diease, and falling away as soon as the acute damage ceases. A disadvantage is that levels in blood samples fall very rapidly in transit and may be quite inaccurate in 24 hours. For this and other reasons, the test is no longer carried out at most laboratories and substitute tests are necessary for acute hepatic damage.

GGT is particularly valuable in detecting chronic liver damage, particularly cirrhosis. It may also rise in pancreatitis. It is a very useful test for ragwort poisoning; and also helps in assessing the degree of chronic change following an acute hepatic lesion.

If SDH is unobtainable, it is best to use *aspartate aminotransferse,* known as AST, AAT or SGOT. Unfortunately, this enzyme is released by acute damage to heart, brain, kidney, and particularly muscle. In fact, the levels of AST produced in serum following acute muscle damage may be very high indeed, reaching 10 000 iu/litre or much more. So, if AST is used as a test for acute liver damage, *CPK* must be used as well to differentiate between liver and muscle pathology.

If SDH, AST (without CPK) or GGT are raised, then it is possibly worth doing SAP and possibly bilirubin. SAP is very useful in hepatic cases where biliary damage has occurred, or where there is obstruction to bile flow, i.e. many cases of chronic liver damage. It should be remembered, however, that alkaline phosphatase is normally raised in young horses with high bone metabolism rates, and allowance must be made for this. Bilirubin assays are not usually a definitive help in the diagnosis of chronic liver disease, because levels can rise during inappetence for whatever cause, and also rise during prehepatic haemolytic disease, during obstinate chronic impactions, and in cases with large traumatic haematoma formations.

(c) *Total and differential serum proteins.* If liver and kidney figures are in normal range, and serum albumin is low, then a protein-losing enteropathy may be present. Low serum albumin levels in the horse, for all practical purposes, occur due to deficient synthesis in the liver or to loss through gut, and if liver figures are normal, then gut function needs investigating. Albumin loss through the kidney, the third possibility, is rare in the horse.

If the investigation so far suggests loss through gut, a *glucose uptake test* may well help, and so may an *intestinal phosphatase* test on serum or plasma.

Serum protein electrophoresis may be very important in the diagnosis of parasitic problems. Use clotted blood, and employ a laboratory which will provide a diagram of the fractionated globulin levels. Gamma globulins rise in tissue wastage, chronic infections, and sometimes in liver disease. But it is very important to remember that alpha 2 and beta globulins rise markedly in migrating strongyle infestations.

(d) *Creatine phosphokinase (CPK)* is a very useful and reasonably specific indication of muscle damage. Its use to decide whether a high AST means liver or muscle damage has been discussed. Remember that CPK is liberated from muscle very easily during exercise or other sudden muscular movement. This is particularly noticeable in young horses. Acute pathological changes in muscle produce spectacular rises in CPK levels, which may reach 10 000 iu/litre plus very easily, as in azoturia.

Remember that blood levels fall very quickly and postal delay may easily produce an inaccurate result.

(e) *Serum chloride levels* give a rough guide to the electrolyte position. Sodium and potassium should also be estimated, but take much longer and add considerably to the cost. Chloride levels should be considered in relation to the PCV, and may well help in assessing the state of dehydration in severe diarrhoea, or in assessing the results of fluid therapy.

Always look at the plasma for signs of hyperlipaemia.

Recently, many laboratories have included *lactate dehydrogenase (LDH)* in their routine. This is a multiple isoenzyme widely distributed in all tissues. The measurement of total enzyme activity is of very little diagnostic value, but the relative increase of one of the five component parts may be of value:

LDH 1 – mostly in heart, brain and testes.

LDH 2 – mostly in non-locomotor muscle, heart, brain, kidney, bone and thyroid.

LDH 3 – mostly in non-locomotor muscle and all major organs.

LDH 4 – mostly in gut, liver and skin.

LDH 5 – mostly in locomotor muscle, gut, liver and skin.

On the whole, these estimations give results too variable and vague to justify the expense.

Lactate and pH values are largely of use in serious colic cases.

(3) Examination of faeces for parasite eggs or larvae, blood and salmonella organisms (where relevant).

(4) Examination of urine, where clinically relevant, or in cases where blood urea is high, for protein, blood, sugars and debris. Always filter equine urine before testing.

(5) In certain cases, dependent as always on clinical findings and on initial laboratory work, further procedures may be required:

(a) *Liver biopsy.*

(b) *Oral glucose uptake* – very useful in malabsorption cases involving the small intestine, e.g. diffuse lymphosarcoma of the gut wall; granulomatous enteritis; and diffuse peritonitis along serous membrane of the gut.

(c) *Bromsulphthalein (BSP) clearance test* for liver function.

(d) *Blood tests for brucellosis* (SAT, CFT and Coomb's tests). *SAT* is significant at +++ in 40 and above. *CFT* is significant at dilutions higher than 1/10. *Coomb's test* is significant at 4 in 160 and above.

(e) *Abdominal paracentesis.*

(f) *Tuberculin test* – somewhat variable in the horse, but nevertheless useful. The technique is as for the cow, but interpretation depends on the appearance and feel of any swelling, rather than upon the measurements.

The routine laboratory scan just described may be summarized as follows:

(1) *Examination of an EDTA sample for the red and white blood cell pictures.*

(2) *Examination of a clotted or heparinized blood (according to the laboratory) for:*

(a) *Urea.*

(b) *SDH and GGT (or AST (plus CPK) and GGT).*

(c) *Total and differential serum proteins.* You may need protein electrophoresis, particularly if strongyle invasion is suspected.

If blood urea is high, do urine analysis.

If SDH, AST (but not CPK) or GGT raised, may do SAP and possibly bilirubin.

If liver and kidney figures alright, but serum albumin is low, then consider protein-losing enteropathy and do glucose uptake and intestinal phosphatase.

(d) CPK.

(e) Cl level, if there is diarrhoea, or in serious colic cases.

(3) *Faecal examination*, e.g. parasite eggs, blood, salmonella.

(4) *In relevant circumstances, you may need:*

(a) *Liver biopsy.*

(b) *BSP clearance.*

(c) *Abdominal paracentesis.*

(d) *Blood samples for brucellosis.*

(e) *The tuberculin test.*

25 Special diagnostic procedures

Stomach tube
Abdominal paracentesis
Liver biopsy
BSP (bromosulphthalein clearance) test
Oral glucose uptake test

Stomach tube

Passage of the stomach tube may be as important for diagnostic purposes as for relieving gastric tympany and fluid distension, for rehydration, for administering medicines, and for feeding in cases unable to chew or swallow.

The modern stomach tube is made of translucent synthetic material and is available in four sizes – large, medium, small and foal. It is very important that the right size be used – if the tube is too wide it causes damage and discomfort, if too narrow it is difficult to pass from the pharynx to the oesophagus, for the horse seems unaware of its presence and makes no attempt to swallow it.

Lay the tube again the horse's head and neck and mark off on it, in ink, the point reached at the nostril when the end of the tube is level with the pharynx, and the point reached at the nostril when the tube is level with the stomach.

Store the tube coiled in the case provided by the manufacturer; the curve so produced is very helpful when passing the tube through the nostrils into the pharynx and then into the oesophagus.

Make sure that the funnel to be used when pouring fluid into the tube, or alternatively, the nozzle of the stomach pump, fits the tube easily, but securely. Do this *before* passing the tube. Warm the business end of the tube either in your hands, or in warm water. Do not leave surplus water in the end of the tube. Lubricate the end well with obstetrical lubricant.

The horse should be backed into a corner to prevent backward movement and restrict sideways movement.

The attendant should stand on the horse's nearside, close to its shoulder, and facing forward. His right arm passes under the horse's chin and up the right side of the head, his hand taking a firm grip over the horse's nasal bones, but not restricting the nostrils. His left hand holds the lead ripe and head collar. Do not attempt to pass a stomach tube in a haltered horse.

In restless horses, the attendant may elect to hold the horse's left ear in his left hand. If a twitch is necessary, the attendant holds the twitch in his left hand. It is important to twist the twitch when applying it in the direction which will not restrict the horse's right nostril.

The operator, assuming he is right handed, stands on the offside of the horse's head. He places his left hand on the horse's nose, and with his first finger or thumb guides the tube downwards into the ventral meatus as his right hand passes the first 6 inches (15 cm) of the tube gently and smoothly into the nostril. It is important that the first 6 inches or so be passed in one movement for this is the part of the procedure which horses resent and if the operator only passes an inch or two at the first movement, it is easy for the horse to shake the tube out again.

The end of the tube should be presented curving downwards so that it follows the ventral meatus and passes smoothly into the pharynx. The rest of the tube should be draped comfortably around the operator's shoulders while the first part of the tube is passed. When the first mark on the tube enters the nostril and the tube is therefore in the pharynx, rotate it through 180° so that the tube end now curves upwards. Advance it until the end of the tube presses upon the back of the pharynx and then tap it on the pharyngeal wall gently several times. Most horses will now swallow it and one feels the peristaltic wave in the oesophagus grip the tube. If a horse refuses to swallow, the tube cannot be passed, but most horses swallow it sooner or later if the operator persists gently and firmly in presenting the tube end to the oesophageal opening. Once the tube is in the oesophagus, push it on smoothly in time with each peristaltic wave. It is often possible to see the movement of the tube in the oesophageal groove in the left side of the neck. If not, it is well worthwhile pressing the fingers of left and right hands firmly together behind the trachea, when, if the finger pressure is sufficient, it is possible to feel the tube. A very useful check when the tube should be about halfway down the neck is to puff sharply into it (not blow – puff) when the bubble of air can be seen distending the oesophagus as it leaves the tube and passes on down. When the tube finally enters the stomach, listen at the distal end of the tube for the churning sounds of gastric movement. Occasionally, eructation will occur and the smell of gas from the stomach will be detected.

If the tube passes down the trachea, the horse will probably cough, breathing sounds will be heard at the end of the tube, and on shaking the trachea with one's hand, the tube can be heard rattling inside it. No significant haemorrhage should occur while passing the tube provided that it is not too wide for the horse's nasal passage, and that neither the operator nor the horse behave roughly. In this connection, it is important to check the tube before use for any abraded areas. If there are any significantly damaged areas, the tube should not be used, as such damage is a frequent cause of haemorrhage.

Liquids given by stomach tube should be slightly warm, i.e. not chillingly cold. A rough guide as to volume is that no more than 1 gallon (4.5 litres) total fluid should be given at any one time to a pony, 1.5 gallons (7 litres) to a riding horse, and 2 gallons (9 litres) to a heavy hunter or cart horse.

Before removing the tube, make sure that it has sufficient time to drain before it is pulled from the oesophagus into the pharynx. It helps to blow down the tube sharply before re-entering the pharynx. Do not pull the tube rapidly out of the oesophagus into the pharynx, for the end may flip upwards and strike the dorsal wall of the pharynx, causing haemorrhage.

It is not proposed to discuss here the passage of the endoscope, except to say that in strange or difficult horses it may be advisable to pass the stomach tube before attempting the endoscope.

Abdominal paracentesis

This should be carried out with head collar or bridle in place. A twitch may be used, if necessary. Clip and cleanse the skin in a 4-inch (10-cm) wide strip between the xiphisternum and the umbilicus. The site of the puncture is at the lowest point of the abdomen, usually about a hand's breadth behind the xiphisternum. Use an 18 or 19 gauge (1.5–2 in) needle. Stand by the horse's left shoulder facing the tail and pass the needle gently through the skin exactly over the midline. Pass the needle on gently through the linea alba into the abdominal cavity. Normally, the horse shows minimal resentment for the linea alba is insensitive, and there is usually no more than slight flinching as the needle penetrates the peritoneal membrane. A certain amount of manipulation and movement of the needle point within the abdomen may be necessary in order to obtain fluid. The more difficult it is to obtain peritoneal fluid, the less likely it is that there is anything abnormal. If the needle ruptures a small blood vessel, it may be withdrawn and a second attempt made about 2 inches (5 cm) anterior or posterior to the first site.

Allow the fluid to run into collection tubes, part into EDTA for a cell count and part should be mixed with 50% ethanol in equal volume for cytology.

Examination of peritoneal fluid may be very useful in determining the severity of a case of acute colic, in the diagnosis of weight loss with or without diarrhoea, in cases which show clinical signs of ascites, and in the investigation of chronic abdominal pain.

The technique is apparently perfectly safe, and no ill effects occur even if penetration of spleen, gut, etc. occurs.

For further details and information regarding laboratory examination of peritoneal fluid, see Bach (1973), Bach and Ricketts (1974) and Ricketts (1983).

Liver biopsy

This procedure is largely used in chronic hepatic disease to assess the degree of irreversible fibrous change. It may be very useful in cases of suspected ragwort poisoning, etc.

Fortunately, most types of liver disease in the horse produce diffuse changes, so one can expect the biopsy sample to be reasonably representative. One of the difficulties associated with this technique in the horse is that there are no biopsy instruments tailored for equine use. A useful instrument which is fairly readily available is the Franklin Liver Needle (152 mm × 12 SWG) supplied by Downs Surgical Ltd (Church Path, Mitcham, Surrey, UK). Recently, a disposable plastic liver biopsy instrument has been designed and marketed.

The procedure is performed as follows: Take a line from the tuber coxae (angle of the haunch) to the point of the elbow, on the right side of the horse. The site is slightly (1 in, 2.5 cm) above this line in the 13th intercostal space (immediately in front of the 14th rib where the intercostal vessels will be safe from damage). There are 18 ribs. Count back from the 18th, ignoring any floating ribs. Prepare an area of some sixteen square inches (40 cm^2), and twitch the horse, if necessary, to infiltrate up to 5 ml of lignocaine HCl at the centre of this area, involving skin and intercostal muscle.

Make a skin incision 0.5 inches (1.25 cm) long, just in front of the rib – pass the trochar and canula into the intercostal muscle. Then, aiming from 10° to 15° backwards, push trochar and canula through the diaphragm, preferably at the point of full expiration, for this will help to involve as little lung as possible. As the instrument passes through the diaphragm, it moves in time with diaphragmatic respiratory movement. Push it on until you feel it impinging on liver. Now, remove the trochar: insert the special split biopsy needle in the canula, and then push the needle firmly into the liver tissue, rotating in the same movement in an attempt to cut out a core of liver tissue. There will be a grating sensation if there are chronic changes present. Withdraw the biopsy needle and place the core of liver into preservative. Put the trochar back into the canula and leave the instrument in place between the ribs until you are satisfied that the minute core of tissue is indeed liver. If unsuccessful, a second attempt may be made in the same intercostal space by altering the direction of the canula slightly. If still unsuccessful, an attempt may be made in the 14th intercostal space. No more than these two secondary attempts may be made on one day. A further attempt may be made in 2 or 3 days' time.

Remove the trochar and canula and suture the skin wound. One suture is sufficient. Do not allow the horse to leave the box for an hour, in order to encourage any haemorrhage to cease and a satisfactory clot to form.

Unfortunate sequelae are very rare, even when samples of lung, diaphragm, kidney, colon wall or contents are obtained in error. Nor does haemorrhage seem to cause problems.

It is, of course, essential that the horse be protected against tetanus, and if there has been an unduly long period of manoeuvring, antibiotics by injection might be a safeguard.

Bromsulphthalein (BSP) clearance test

The ability of the liver to clear BSP from the circulation may be helpful in assessing liver function.

Collect a heparinized sample of blood from the jugular vein (control). Inject 1 g dye into the jugular vein using a heparinized needle (size 18 SWG can be used flushed out in heparin solution). Withdraw needle.

Using a new needle (heparinized) be ready to collect the first sample 2 minutes after injection. Control the flow of blood from the needle by using a thumb.

Collect samples every 2 minutes thereafter until 10 minutes and then two further samples at 12 and 15 minutes.

For determination of the BSP concentrations, a standard solution is made by taking 1 ml of solution from the bottle or ampoule of BSP used for injection and making up to 1 litre with water in a volumetric flask. An aliquot of this standard solution (50 µg/ml) and of the plasmas from each of the blood samples are mixed with an equal volume of N/10 sodium hydroxide and read in the colorimeter with a green filter.

The BSP concentration for each plasma is:

$$\frac{\text{Test control}}{\text{Standard}} \times 50\,\mu g/ml$$

This is plotted on two-cycle semi-log. paper against time, time being plotted on the linear scale and concentration on the logarithmic scale. A linear plot should result, and the time for the concentration to fall to half its value ($T_{1/2}$) can be calculated. The samples may be sent by post to the laboratory, who will check them and prepare the graph. *The normal half-time is 2.5 minutes. A clearance time in excess of 3 minutes indicates functional liver deficiency.*

Oral glucose uptake test

A very useful indication of the efficiency of the small intestine in the absorption of nutrients.

The horse is starved overnight and kept on peat or other inedible bedding. Water is allowed until the beginning of the test.

Anhydrous glucose (1.0 g/kg body weight) or glucose monohydrate (1.1 g/kg body weight) is given by stomach tube in 20% solution in warm water; having infiltrated lignocaine over the jugular vein and taken a pretest blood sample in oxalate-fluoride for a fasting glucose estimate.

Further samples are taken at 30, 60, 90, 120 and 180 minutes after dosing.

In order to save time and money, two samples only may be taken at 60 and 120 minutes after dosing.

In normal horses, the level at 120 minutes is approximately double the fasting level. This level falls back to normal in a further 4 hours.

In complete malabsorption cases, the resting glucose does not rise at all, and diagnosis and prognosis are clear cut.

Unfortunately, an intermediate picture may occur in which the glucose level rises in the 2-hour period, but by no means reaches the normal level. Such cases of relative malabsorption may, or may not, recover, and one can only give supportive treatment and allow time in the hope that recovery will ensue.

A further glucose uptake test in a few weeks may help to assess progress.

References

Bach, L. G. (1973) Exfoliative cytology of peritoneal fluid in the horse. In *The Veterinary Annual* (eds C. S. Grunsell and F. W. G. Hill), Wright, Bristol, pp. 102–109

Bach, L. G. and Ricketts, S. W. (1974) Paracentesis as an aid to the diagnosis of abdominal disease in the horse. *Equine Veterinary Journal*, **6** (3), 116–121

Ricketts, S. W. (1983) Technique of paracentesis abdominis (peritoneal tap) in the horse. *Equine Veterinary Journal*, **15** (3), 288–289

Roberts, M. C. and Hill, F. W. G. (1973) The oral glucose tolerance test. *Equine Veterinary Journal*, **5** (4), 171

Further reading

Allen, W. E. (1988) *Fertility and Obstetrics in the Horse*, Blackwell Scientific, Oxford

Brown, C. M. (1989) *Problems in Equine Medicine*, Lea & Febiger, Philadelphia

Denny, H. R. (1989) *Treatment of Equine Fractures*, Wright, London

Hickman, J. (ed.) (1985, 1986) *Equine Surgery and Medicine*, vols 1, 2 (Animal Care, Health and Welfare Series), Academic, London

Hickman, J. (ed.) (1984) *Horse Management* (Animal Care, Health and Welfare Series), Academic, London

Johnston, A. M. (1986) *Equine Medical Disorders* (Library of Veterinary Practice), Blackwell Scientific, Oxford

Rossdale, P. D. and Ricketts, S. W. (1980) *Equine Stud Farm Medicine*, 2nd edn, Baillière Tindall, London

Stashak, Ted S. (1987) *Adams' Lameness in Horses*, 4th edn, Lea & Febiger, Philadelphia

Amstutz, H. E., McAllister, E. S. and Pratt, P. W. (eds) (1982) *Equine Medicine and Surgery*, American Veterinary Publications

It is not suggested that the books listed above should be bought in the first instance, but that they should be obtained from time to time from the library of the Royal College of Veterinary Surgeons, the reader's practice library, or from other suitable libraries. It is also recommended that the *Equine Veterinary Journal*, *Equine Veterinary Education* and *In Practice* should be checked whenever possible for papers of particular interest.

Index

Abcess, 127
Abdominal catastrophe, 19–22
Abdominal lymphosarcoma, 32–35
Abdominal pain
  diseases simulating, 29–30
  see also Colic
Abdominal paracentesis, 182–183
Acepromazine in treatment of colic, 12
Acne, 114
Actinobacillus equuli, 154
Acute cardiac failure, 122
Acute renal failure, 62
Acute venous congestion of lungs, 80
Adenovirus, 69
Allergic and anaphylactic conditions,
  93–96
Anaemia, 59
Anthrax, 20, 123, 126
  diarrhoea in, 40
Ascariasis, 157
Aspartate aminotransferase,
  measurement of, 174
Aspergillus growth in gut, 46
Atresia ani, 164
Atresia coli, 164
Atrial fibrillation, 147–148
Avian tuberculosis of large gut, 45–46,
  51
'Avonmouth' disease, 109–110
Azoturia, 98–99

Bacillus piliformis, 161
Belching, 16–17
Biliary tract obstruction, 57–59
  and skin lesions, 117
Blood vessels, lymphosarcoma
  involving, 36
Bone marrow, lymphosarcoma
  involving, 36
Botulism, 83–84, 124
Bracken poisoning, 131
Brain, space-occupying lesions in,
  133–134
Bromsulphthalein clearance test, 176,
  184–185
Brucellosis, 127–128

Campylobacter spp., 156
Carcinomas, 116
Cardiac septal defects, 164
Cataract, 140–141
Cereal overeating, 44
Cerebellar hypoplasia, 165
'Choke', 85
Cholelithiasis, 58
Chronic interstitial nephritis, 62
Chronic parasitic colitis, 45
Chronic parasitic ulcerative colitis,
  44–45
Chronic pulmonary disease, 70–72, 88
Cirrhosis, *see* Liver disease, chronic
Clinical attitude, 2
Clinician's approach, 2–3
  lameness, 104–108
Clostridial enterotoxaemia, 42
Clostridium difficile, 156
Clostridium perfringens, 42, 156
Clostridium septique, 124
Clostridium welchii, 42, 156
Colic, 9–30
  abdominal examination per rectum,
    15
  causes, 27–28
  chronic, 27–29
    laboratory examinations in, 171
  diagnosis and managment, 10–11,
    29
  faecal passage, 15–16
  in foal, 159–160
  gastric, 22–23
  gastric filling, belching, 'vomiting',
    16–17
  generalized muscular tremors in, 15
  intestinal, 23–24
  laboratory aids to assessment of
    critical case, 17, 170
  mucous membranes in, 14
  pulse rate and character in, 13–14
  relief of, 11–13
  respiratory pattern in, 14–15
Combined immunodeficiency, 165
Congenital conditions of foal, 163–166
Contracted flexor tendons, 164
Cornea, examination of, 140

Corynebacterium equi, 156, 157–158
Coughing, 65–74
    chronic pulmonary disease, 70–72
    equine influenza, 67–68
    nasopharyngeal lymphoid
        hyperplasia, 73–74
    parasitic bronchitis, 73
    pollen allergy, 73
    rhinitis, 67
    rhinopneumonitis, 68–69
    strangles, 66–67
    viral conditions, 69–70
Cranial nerve damage, 82
Creatine phosphokinase,
    measurement of, 175
Cushing's disease, 117
Cystitis, 63

Degenerative changes, 62
Dermatophilus congolense infection, 113
Description, 5
Diagnosis
    colic, 10–11
    wasting, 48–49
Diagnostic procedures, 179–186
Diaphragmatic hernia, 76–77
Diarrhoea, 39–46, 50–51
    acute, 40–44
    chronic, 44–46
    in foal, 155–157
    oestral, 157
Dysphagia, 81–86, 89
    botulism, 83–84
    'choke', 85
    cranial nerve damage, 82
    grass sickness, 85–86
    guttural pouch, 84
    hyperlipaemia, 83
    lead poisoning, 83
    mouth, lips, teeth, 82
    paralysis of pharyngeal nerve,
        84–85
    pharyngitis, 84
    polymyositis, 83
    tetanus, 82
    thoracic lymphosarcoma, 83
Dyspnoea, 75–80
    acute anaphylactic shock, 79
    acute venous congestion of lungs,
        80
    conditions simulating, 80
    diaphragmatic hernia, 76–77
    Marie's disease, 79
    pleurisy, pleural effusion, 'transit
        fever', stress, 77
    pneumonia, 77–78
    thoracic lymphosarcoma, 78–79
    tuberculosis, 79

Ehlers–Danlos syndrome, 116–117
Electrocution, 122
Endocarditis, 127
    chronic vegetative, 148
Enteritis, acute, 21, 123
Enteroliths, 25–26
Entropion in foal, 139–140, 163
Epileptiform fits, 135
Equine herpes virus
    type 1, 135, 158
    type 2, 69, 158
Equine influenza, 67–68
Examination, 5–8, 144–147
Eye, 137–142
    cataract, 140–141
    corneal problems, 140
    entropion, 139–140
    excessive lacrimation, 139
    foreign bodies in, 138–139
    injuries to periorbital region and
        eyelids, 138
    neoplasms in, 139
    protrusion of third eyelid, 139
    retinal haemorrhage, 142
    uveitis, 141–142

Faecal examination, 176
Faecal passage, 15–16
Falling horse, 134–135
Flunixin meglamine in treatment of
    colic, 12
Foal, diseases of, 151–166
    'colic' syndromes, 159–160
    congenital conditions, 163–166
    diarrhoea, 155–157
    haemolytic disease of newborn foal,
        160–161
    hepatitis, 161–162
    neonatal infections, 154–155
    neurological conditions, 158–159
    orthopaedic conditions, 160
    respiratory conditions, 157–158
    steatitis, polymyositis and
        hyperlipaemia, 162–163
    tetanus, 162
Food impaction, see Intestinal
    impaction
Foreign bodies in eye, 138–139
Fungal growth in gut, 46

Gallstones, 58
Gamma glutamyl transferase
    in biliary tract obstruction, 57
    measurement of, 174
Gastric colic, 22–23
Gastric filling, 16–17
Granulomatous colitis, 45, 51

Grass sickness, 19–20, 33, 51, 85–86
  chronic, and diarrhoea, 46
  peracute, 124
Greasy heel, 117
Guttural pouch
  disease, 88
  tympany, 84, 164

Haematuria, 63–64
Haemoglobinuria, 64
Haemolytic disease of newborn foal,
    160–161
Haemorrhage, 122
  retinal, 142
Harvest mites, 113
Head flicking, 136
Heart disease, 143–149
  atrial fibrillation, 147–148
  cardiac hypertrophy, 148
  chronic, and wasting, 52
  chronic vegetative endocarditis, 148
  clinical examination, 144–147
  congenital cardiac problems, 149
  myocarditis, 149
  pericarditis, 148–149
Heat stroke, 131–132
Hepatic disease, see Liver disease
Hepatic encephalopathy, 131
Hepatitis, 161–162
Hernia
  scrotal/inguinal in foal, 164
  umbilical in foal, 164–165
History, 4–5
Horner's syndrome, 139
Hyoscine, in treatment of colic, 12
Hyperkeratosis of ear pinna, 114
Hyperlipaemia, 43–44, 56, 83
  in foal, 162
Hypocalcaemia, 124, 130

Intestinal colic, 23–24
  flatulent or tympanitic, 23–24
    in foal, 159
  spasmodic, 23
Intestinal impaction, 24–27
Intussusception, 159

Jaundice, 58–59

Kidney disease, chronic, and wasting,
    52

Laboratory examinations, 7–8,
    167–177
  aspartate aminotransferase, 174
  blood urea, 173
  bromsulphthalein clearance test,
    176, 184–185

Laboratory examinations (cont.)
  in colic, 17
  creatine phosphokinase, 175
  faecal examination, 176
  gamma glutamyl transferase, 174
  lactate dehydrogenase, 175–176
  normal haematological ranges, 173
  oral glucose uptake, 176, 185
  red cells, 171–172
  serum chloride levels, 175
  sorbitol dehydrogenase, 174
  total and differential serum
      proteins, 174–175
  tuberculin test, 176
  white cells, 172–173
Lactate dehydrogenase, measurement
    of, 175–176
Lameness, 103–110
  'Avonmouth' disease, 109–110
  clinical approach, 104–108
  sporadic lymphangitis, 108–109
  weanling disease, 109
Laminitis, 127
Lead poisoning, 83, 92, 109–110, 131
Lethargy, 59
Lice, 112
Lightning strike, 122
Listeriosis, 133
Liver biopsy, 183–184
Liver disease, 53–59
  acute, 54–56
  chronic, 56–57
    anaemia, lethargy and poor
        performance, 59
    cholelithiasis, 58
    and diarrhoea, 46
    jaundice, 58–59
    pancreatic lesions causing biliary
        tract obstruction, 57–59
    and wasting, 51
  secondary, 56
Louping-ill, 132–133
Lungworm disease, 73
Lymph nodes, lymphosarcoma
    involving, 37
Lymphoid tissue, lymphosarcoma
    involving, 37
Lymphosarcoma, 31–37, 51
  abdominal, 32–35
    differential diagnosis, 35
  diffuse infiltration of wall of large
      gut, 45
  generalized, 36–37
  of skin, 37
  thoracic, 35–36, 78–79, 83

Mange, 112–113
Marie's disease, 79

Mastication, conditions interfering with, 49–50
Mastitis, 120
Meconium retention, 159
Melanoma, 115
Metamizole in treatment of colic, 12
Missed ventricular beats, 134
Mouth, injuries to, 92
Mucous membranes in colic, 14
Muscular dystrophy, 83, 99–101, 124
Muscular problems, 97–101
    azoturia, 98–99
    polymyositis, 83, 99–101, 124
    'tied-up' syndrome, 98
Muscular tremors in colic, 15
Myocarditis, 149
Myoglobinuria, 64

Narcolepsy, 134
Nasal discharge, 87–89
Nasopharyngeal lymphoid hyperplasia, 73–74
Necrobiosis, 116
Neonatal maladjustment syndromes, 158–159
Neoplasia, 115–116
    of eye, 139
Nervous symptoms, diseases producing, 129–136
    botulism, 132
    bracken poisoning, 131
    falling horse, 134–135
    in foal, 158–159
    heat stroke, 131–132
    hepatic encephalopathy, 131
    hypocalcaemia, 130
    lead poisoning, 131
    listeriosis, 133
    localized nervous syndromes, 135–136
    louping-ill, 132–133
    polymyositis, 132
    rabies, 133
    space-occupying lesions in the brain, 133–134
    synchronous diaphragmatic flutter, 130–131
    tetanus, 132
    transit tetany, 130
    uraemia, 131
Neuritis of cauda equina, 136
Nodular disease, 116
Nutrition and diarrhoea, 44

Oral glucose uptake test, 176, 185
Organophosphorus poisoning, 21, 92
    and diarrhoea, 43
Orthopaedic conditions of foals, 160
Oxyuris equi, 114

Pain in colic, 14
Pancreatic lesions causing biliary tract obstruction, 57–59
Papilloma, 115
Parafilaria multipapillosa, 114
Parasites and bacteria causing skin diseases, 112–115
Parasitic bronchitis, 73
Peracute disease, 123–124
Pericarditis, 148–149
Peritonitis, 43, 51
Pervious urachus, 164
Pethidine, in treatment of colic, 12
Pharyngeal nerve paralysis, 84–85
Pharyngitis, 84
Phenylbutazone, prolonged therapy, and diarrhoea, 46
Plant hepatotoxins, 54
Pleural effusion, 77
Pleurisy, 77
Pneumonia, 126
Pollen allergy, 73
Polymyositis, 83, 99–101, 124
    in foal, 162–163
Poor performance, 59
Preliminary inspection, 5
Pulse rate and character in colic, 13–14
Purpura haemorrhagica, 21–22, 43, 94–95, 123
Pyelonephritis, 62
Pyosepticaemia, 155
Pyrexia of unknown origin, 125–128

Rabies, 133
Rectal examination, 15
Redwater, 63–64
Redworm infestation, 16, 29, 51
Reovirus, 69
Respiratory disease
    coughing, see Coughing
    dyspnoea, see Dyspnoea
    in foal, 157–158
Respiratory pattern in colic, 14–15
Retinal haemorrhage, 142
Rhinitis, 67
Rhinopneumonitis, 68–69
Rhododendron poisoning, 43, 92
Ringworm, 112
Ruptured bladder, 159–160

Salivation, 91–92
Salmonella enteritidis, 21, 40
Salmonella indiana, 21, 40, 50
Salmonella newport, 21, 40
Salmonella typhimurium, 21, 40, 156

Salmonellosis
  acute, 40–42
  chronic, 46, 50
Sarcoids, 115
Septicaemia, 126
  in foal
    coliform, 155
    streptococcal, 155
Serum alkaline phosphatase in biliary
    tract obstruction, 57
Skin diseases, 111–117
  allergic conditions, 95, 115
  biliary obstruction, 117
  Cushing's disease, 117
  Ehlers–Danlos syndrome, 116–117
  greasy heel, 117
  lymphosarcoma, 37, 116
  neoplasia, 115–116
  nodular disease, 116
  parasites and bacteria, 112–115
  vitiligo, 116
'Sleepy foal' disease, 154
Sorbitol dehyrogenase, measurement
    of, 174
Sporadic lymphangitis, 108–109
Steatitis, 163
Stomach tube, 180–182
Strangles, 66–67
Streptococcus equi, 43
Streptococcus zooepidemicus, 120
Stress, 77
Strongylus vulgaris, 44, 156, 160
Sudden death and 'found dead'
    syndromes, 122
Superpurgation, 40
Swallowing, conditions interfering
    with, 49–50
Sweet-itch, 96
Synchronous diaphragmatic flutter,
    130–131

Tetanus, 82, 132
  in foal, 162
Thoracic lesions, 35–36
'Tied-up' syndrome, 98
Torsion of small intestine, 123
'Transit fever', 77
Transit tetany, 124, 130
Tuberculin test, 176
Tuberculosis, 79
Tympany
  gastric, 22–23
  guttural pouch, 164
  intestinal, 23–24
    in foal, 159
Tyzzer's disease, 161–162

Udder, 119–120
Upper respiratory tract infections, 88
Uraemia, 131
Urea, measurement of, 173
Urinary symptoms, diseases
    producing, 61–64
  acute renal failure, 62
  chronic interstitial nephritis, 62
  cystitis, 63
  degenerative changes, 62
  pyelonephritis, 62
  redwater, 63–64
  urolithiasis, 63
Urolithiasis, 63
Urticaria, 95
Uveitis, 141–142

Viraemia, 128
Viral ataxia, 158
Viral hepatitis, 54–56
Viruses
  diarrhoea as complication of, 43
  and liver disease, 54–55
Vitiligo, 116
Volvulus, 159
Vomiting, 16–17
  gross, 19–20

Warbles, 114–115
Wasting, 47–52
  chronic heart conditions, 52
  chronic kidney conditions, 52
  chronic liver disease, 51
  conditions causing persistent low-
      grade pain, 49
  conditions interfering with
      intestinal function, 50–51
  conditions interfering with
      mastication and/or swallowing,
      49–50
  diagnosis, 48–49
  laboratory examination in, 171
  miscellaneous causes, 52
Water dropwort, 122
Weanling disease, 109
Wobbler syndrome, 135, 165–166
Wound gas gangrene, 124

Yew poisoning, 122

Zinc poisoning, 109–110